Baby & Child Emergency First Aid Handbook

Simple Step-By-Step Instructions for the Most Common Childhood Emergencies

Edited by Mitchell J. Einzig, M.D.

Meadowbrook Press
Distributed by Simon & Schuster
New York

Distributed in the U.K. by
Chris Lloyd Sales and Marketing

Library of Congress Cataloging-in-Publication Data

Baby & child emergency first aid handbook: simple step-by-step
  instructions for the most common childhood emergencies / edited by
  Mitchell J. Einzig; illustrated by Nancy Lynch.
        p.   cm.
     Includes index.
     ISBN 0-88166-195-3
     1.   Pediatric emergencies—Handbooks, manuals, etc. 2.   First aid
in illness and injury—Handbooks, manuals, etc.   I. Einzig,
Mitchell J.   II. Title: Baby and child emergency first aid handbook.
  RJ370.B3   1992
  618.92'00252—dc20   92-28339
                                                                       CIP

Simon & Schuster Ordering # 0-671-79204-0

Writer and Development Editor: Kerstin Gorham
Copy Editor: Jane Strovas
Editorial Director: Jay Johnson
Production Coordinator: Matthew Thurber
Desktop Coordinator: Jon C. Wright
Cover and Page Design: Tabor Harlow
Cover and Interior Art: Nancy Lynch

The contents of this book have been reviewed and checked for accuracy and appropriateness of
application by medical professionals. However, the editors and publisher disclaim all
responsibility arising from any adverse effects or results that occur or might occur as a result of
the inappropriate application of any of the information contained in this book. If you have any
questions or concerns about the appropriateness or application of the treatments described in
this book, consult your health-care professional. Further, the views expressed in this book are
not necessarily the views of the Minneapolis Children's Medical Center or the University of
Minnesota.

Published by Meadowbrook Press, 18318 Minnetonka Boulevard, Deephaven, MN 55391.

BOOK TRADE DISTRIBUTION by Simon & Schuster, a division of Simon and Schuster, Inc.,
1230 Avenue of the Americas, New York, NY 10020.

First published in the U.K. 1992.
DISTRIBUTED IN THE U.K. AND IRELAND by Chris Lloyd Sales and Marketing,
P.O. Box 327, Poole, Dorset BH15 2RG.

93 94 95 96 97 98   6 5 4 3 2 1

Printed in the United States of America

A **FREE** Meadowbrook Press catalog is available upon request.
Call Toll-Free at 1-800-338-2232.

Contents iii

iv Contents

As a father and pediatrician, I know that nothing is more frightening than when your child experiences a medical emergency. Other than calling an emergency number, parents are often unsure of what to do. With most emergencies, however, there are steps you can take to help your child before medical help is available. The *Baby & Child Emergency First Aid Handbook* is designed to provide you with those first aid steps that sometimes save lives.

Most emergency first aid books currently available overwhelm you with excessive information that is often impractical and poorly organized. The illustrations in these books often do not clearly relate to the text and may look stark and frightening.

Based on my years of experience in pediatrics, I have selected the most common childhood emergencies and provided you with directions for essential, practical first aid treatment.

This book is designed to be easily read during an emergency. Use the index on the front or back cover (or the contents on pages iii–iv) to look up the specific topic you need. On the page indicated, you'll find information required before you begin first aid, including instructions on when to get professional help, which signs and symptoms to monitor, and what *not* to do. The first aid steps are clearly numbered, written in large type, and accompanied by reassuring illustrations.

When you get this book, first fill out the Parents' Emergency Information Page at the back of the book so the phone numbers you need will be readily at hand. It is also a good idea to have the emergency first aid supplies listed on page vi. Next, read through the emergency first aid treatment entries to familiarize yourself with basic information about specific emergencies. Be sure to keep the book in an easily accessible location. Finally, take a basic course in CPR (cardiopulmonary resuscitation) if you have not already done so, or retake it if you have not done so in the last one to two years. The techniques for CPR are most effectively and safely learned and reviewed through personal instruction and supervised practice.

I hope you never have occasion to use this book. But if you do, it will help you take safe, effective action in an emergency until professional help is available. Good luck to you and your family.

vi First Aid Supplies

Keep the following supplies out of children's reach, but easily accessible in an emergency.

- **Adhesive bandages: assorted sizes**
- **Adhesive tape: ½ to 1 inch (1¼ to 2½ cm) wide**
- **Antibiotic ointment**
- **Antihistamines (over-the-counter)**
- **Antiseptic wipes or solution**
- **Calamine lotion**
- **Cool-mist vaporizer**
- **Cotton balls**
- **Cotton swabs**
- **Elastic bandages**
- **Heating pad**
- **Hot-water bottle**
- **Pain-relieving tablets or liquid (acetaminophen or paracetamol)**
- **Scissors with blunt tips**
- **Sterile eye wash**
- **Sterile gauze bandages and pads**
- **Syrup of ipecac**
- **Thermometer (oral or rectal)**
- **Triangular bandages and safety pins**
- **Tweezers (round-ended)**

A splint is used to immobilize an injured body part and protect it from further injury. In general, don't try to move or reposition a fractured bone or dislocated joint. Always immobilize it in the position in which it was found. Follow these general steps when splinting a body part.

1. Use something rigid and flat for the splint, such as a board, ruler, stick, or rolled-up magazine or newspaper. You can also use a pillow or blanket, or in some cases another body part, such as a leg or finger.

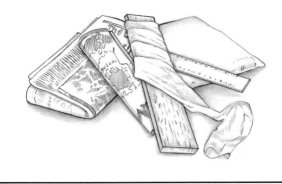

2. If the splint is hard and rigid, pad it with cloths or towels before attaching it.

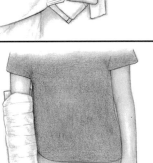

3. Be certain the splint extends to the joints above and below a fracture.

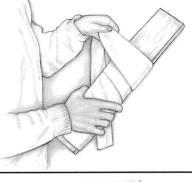

4. Tie the splint to the injured part with cloth strips, tape, belts, or neckties. Be careful not to attach the splint too tightly; if the fingers or toes become pale and cool, loosen the splint. Don't let knots press against the injured area.

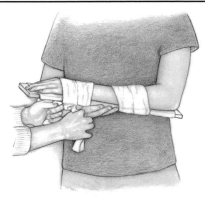

A sling is used to immobilize an injured shoulder, collarbone, or forearm and place it in a position of comfort. Follow these general steps when making a sling.

1. **Make a triangular sling by folding a square yard of cloth diagonally, or improvise by using an item of clothing.**

   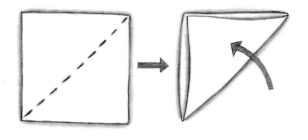

2. **Have your child support her injured arm while you slip the sling under the arm, as shown.**

3. **Fold the cloth around the arm and pull the edges up over your child's shoulders.**

   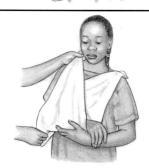

4. **Tie a knot on the side of your child's neck. Pin up the extra cloth at her elbow.**

   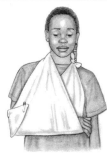

5. **With some injuries, to decrease mobility, tie the sling to your child's body with another piece of cloth, knotting the cloth on the uninjured side.**

   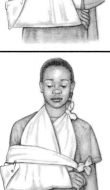

Emergency
First Aid
Treatment

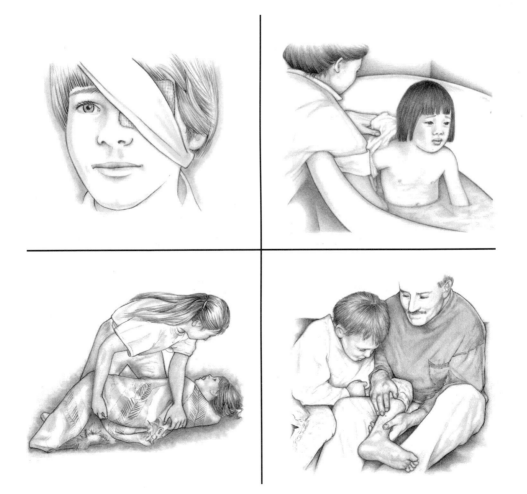

SIGNS & SYMPTOMS

- Rash with or without hives, lip swelling, stuffy nose; if more severe, abdominal pain, vomiting, diarrhea, wheezing; if very severe, shock.

WHAT YOU NEED TO KNOW

- An allergy is a sensitivity to a specific substance (e.g., food, poison ivy, bee sting venom).
- Most severe reactions occur relatively soon after contact with or ingestion of a foreign substance.
- The majority of reactions are relatively mild and can be treated at home.

WHEN TO GET PROFESSIONAL HELP

- If your child has difficulty breathing, call your local emergency number.
- If you think your child is having an allergic reaction, call your doctor.

WHAT TO CHECK

- Observe your child's breathing and check the pulse. If needed, begin CPR:

  If your child is under 1 year old, see page 12—BREATHING/CARDIAC EMERGENCY, For Infant Under 1 Year.

  If your child is 1 to 8 years old, see page 16—BREATHING/CARDIAC EMERGENCY, For Child Age 1–8 Years.

  If your child is over 8 years old, see page 20—BREATHING/CARDIAC EMERGENCY, For Child Over 8 Years.

1. Calm and reassure your child; anxiety can increase the severity of a reaction.

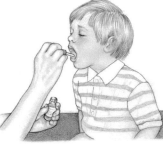

2. If the reaction is mild, give your child over-the-counter antihistamines.

Follow the dosage recommended on the package label.

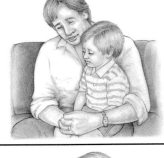

3. If your child has an itchy rash, apply calamine lotion or cool compresses to alleviate itching.

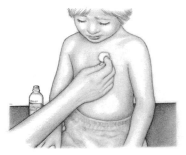

2 Amputation

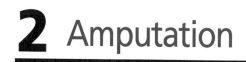

WHAT YOU NEED TO KNOW

- Remain calm; severed parts often can be surgically reattached.

WHEN TO GET PROFESSIONAL HELP

- If your child severs a limb, finger, or toe, call your local emergency number immediately.

1. Reassure and comfort your child.

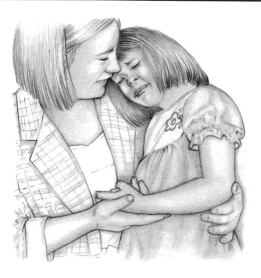

2. If the stump is bleeding, apply direct pressure with a clean, dry cloth.

Maintain firm but gentle pressure for 5 to 10 minutes or until the bleeding subsides. If blood soaks through the cloth, don't remove it; you may loosen the clot. Place another cloth over the first one.

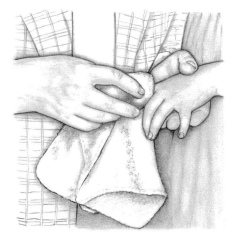

CONTINUED ON NEXT PAGE |||⟩

3. When the bleeding has subsided, even if the wound is still oozing, cover the stump with a clean cloth.

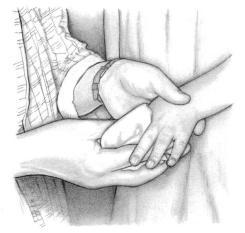

4. If possible, raise the injured area above heart level to reduce bleeding.

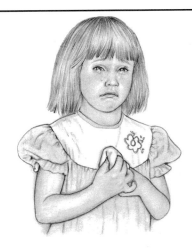

5. Wrap the severed part in a clean, damp cloth, place it in a sealed plastic bag, and immerse the bag in cold water.

Don't put the severed part directly on ice. If cold water is not available, keep the part away from heat. Save it for the emergency personnel or take it with you to the hospital.

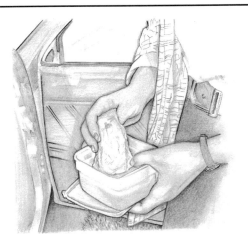

4 Asthma

- Coughing and wheezing, which may progress to severe difficulty breathing.

- If your child (a) is experiencing asthma for the first time, (b) does not respond to his prescribed treatment, or (c) has a temperature over 102°F (39°C), call your doctor.

1. Calm and reassure your child; anxiety can increase the severity of asthma.

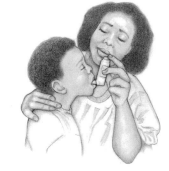

2. Give your child prescribed medication.

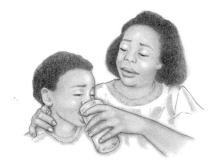

3. Give your child clear liquids.

4. Have your child rest in a well-ventilated room.

If he has trouble breathing while lying down, have him sit up.

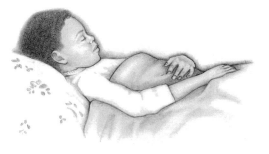

WHAT YOU NEED TO KNOW

- Puncture wounds—which are common with cat and human bites—pose the highest risk of infection.

WHAT TO CHECK

- Determine whether your child's immunizations are current.

- Observe the animal's behavior. Rabies are a particular concern with bats, skunks (North America only), foxes, and stray cats and dogs. Rabies are not a concern with squirrels, rabbits, and other rodents.

WHEN TO GET PROFESSIONAL HELP

- If your child has multiple bites and/or severe bleeding, call your local emergency number.

- If the bite broke the skin, call your doctor.

DON'TS

- Don't clean the bite with alcohol or hydrogen peroxide, which may injure normal tissue.

1. If the bite is bleeding profusely, apply direct pressure with a clean, dry cloth until the bleeding subsides.

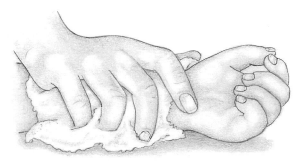

2. Wash the bite with soap and lukewarm running water for 3 to 5 minutes and pat dry.

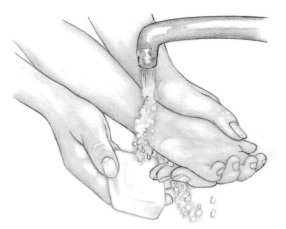

CONTINUED ON NEXT PAGE ⫸

3. **Cover the bite with a clean dressing.**

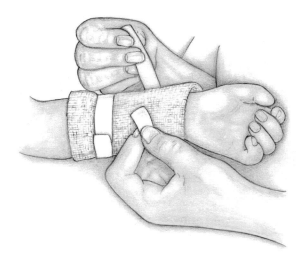

4. **Over the next 24 to 48 hours, observe the bite for signs of infection (increasing redness, swelling, and pain).**

If the bite becomes infected, call your doctor or take your child to an emergency facility.

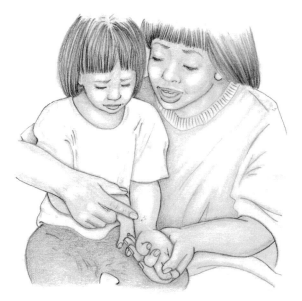

SIGNS & SYMPTOMS

- A *mild reaction* may include pain, redness, and 1 to 2 inches (2½ to 5 cm) of swelling around the bite, usually lasting less than 24 to 48 hours.

- A *severe reaction* may include a rash with or without itching and hives, coughing, wheezing, and difficulty breathing.

WHAT YOU NEED TO KNOW

- Severe allergic reactions to bee stings are very uncommon and usually occur shortly after the sting.

WHAT TO CHECK

- Observe your child's breathing and check the pulse. If needed, begin CPR:

  If your child is under 1 year old, see page 12—BREATHING/CARDIAC EMERGENCY, For Infant Under 1 Year.

  If your child is 1 to 8 years old, see page 16—BREATHING/CARDIAC EMERGENCY, For Child Age 1–8 Years.

  If your child is over 8 years old, see page 20—BREATHING/CARDIAC EMERGENCY, For Child Over 8 Years.

WHEN TO GET PROFESSIONAL HELP

- If your child has difficulty breathing, call your local emergency number.

- If your child has a rash, call your doctor.

1. If the sting is from a honey bee, remove the stinger.

If the stinger is difficult to grasp, try to ease it out by gently scraping against the stinger with a fingernail, credit card, or table knife. Don't try to squeeze it with tweezers. If it is too deep to remove, call your doctor for instructions.

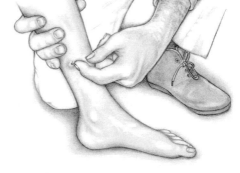

2. Wash the site with soap and lukewarm water.

If calamine lotion is available, dab some on the affected area to reduce discomfort.

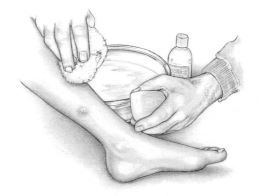

CONTINUED ON NEXT PAGE ||||⮕

3. **Cover the site with a clean, cold compress or a clean, moist dressing to reduce swelling and discomfort.**

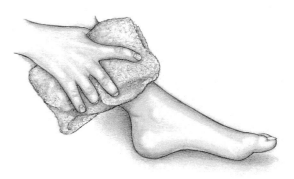

4. **Over the next 24 to 48 hours, observe the site for signs of infection (increasing redness, swelling, and pain).**

If the site becomes infected, call your doctor or take your child to an emergency room.

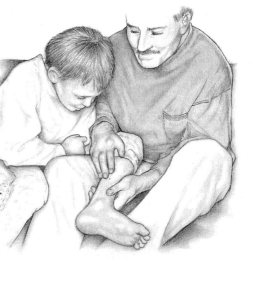

SIGNS & SYMPTOMS

- One or two fang marks in the skin; burning, swelling, pain, or discoloration. *If venom enters the bloodstream,* nausea and vomiting may occur and progress to shock (rapid, shallow breathing; weak, rapid pulse).

WHEN TO GET PROFESSIONAL HELP

- If the bite is from a poisonous snake, call your local emergency number, or take your child to a hospital, immediately. Time is of the essence. If possible, call the hospital so antivenin can be ready when you arrive.

WHAT TO CHECK

- Observe your child's breathing and check the pulse. If necessary, begin CPR:

  If your child is under 1 year old, see page 12—BREATHING/CARDIAC EMERGENCY, For Infant Under 1 Year.

  If your child is 1 to 8 years old, see page 16—BREATHING/CARDIAC EMERGENCY, For Child Age 1–8 Years.

  If your child is over 8 years old, see page 20—BREATHING/CARDIAC EMERGENCY, For Child Over 8 Years.

DON'TS

- Don't give your child anything by mouth.

- Don't apply a tourniquet, make incisions in the wound, or suction the venom; doing so may cause more harm than good.

---

1. Keep your child calm, restrict her movement, and keep the affected area below heart level to reduce the flow of venom.

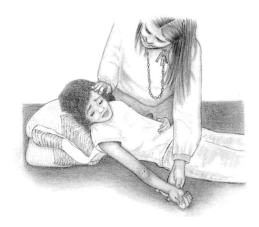

---

2. Cover the bite with a clean, cool compress or a clean, moist dressing to reduce swelling and discomfort.

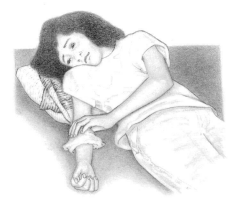

10 Bleeding

WHAT YOU NEED TO KNOW

- Direct pressure will stop most bleeding.

- Bleeding from the scalp is not always as serious as it seems; a small cut can appear to bleed profusely.

WHAT TO CHECK

- If the bleeding cannot be controlled, observe your child for shock. If the child becomes dizzy or faint and/or develops pale, cool, clammy skin; rapid, shallow breathing; and a weak, rapid pulse, continue to treat the bleeding and turn to page 80—SHOCK.

WHEN TO GET PROFESSIONAL HELP

- If the bleeding can't be controlled or is associated with a serious injury, call your local emergency number.

- If you think the wound might need stitches, or if embedded gravel or dirt cannot be removed easily with gentle cleaning, take your child to an emergency facility. Prompt treatment is important to avoid contamination.

DON'TS

- Don't apply a tourniquet to control bleeding; doing so may cause more harm than good.

1. Calm and reassure your child.

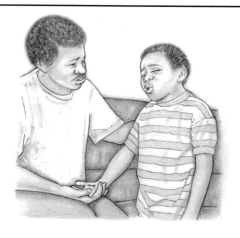

2. Apply direct pressure to the wound with a clean, dry cloth.

Maintain firm but gentle pressure for 5 to 10 minutes or until the bleeding subsides. If blood soaks through the cloth, don't remove it; you may loosen the clot. Place another cloth over the first one.

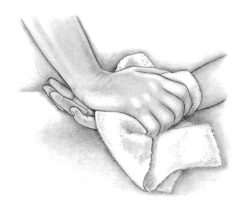

CONTINUED ON NEXT PAGE ‖‖‖➡

3. **If the wound is superficial, wash it with soap and warm water and pat dry.**

Don't wash a wound that is deep or bleeding profusely. If you are unsure about the seriousness of the wound, call your doctor.

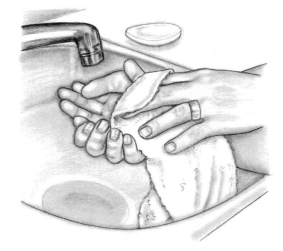

4. **When the bleeding has subsided, even if the wound is still oozing, place a clean dressing over the wound.**

Bandage the dressing firmly, but not so tightly that the child's skin beyond the wound becomes pale and cool, which indicates that the circulation is cut off.

WHAT YOU NEED TO KNOW

- The procedures for CPR (cardiopulmonary resuscitation) described below are not a substitute for CPR training; they are performed most effectively and safely by those trained in CPR.

- If choking is the cause of breathing difficulty, follow the procedures on page 30—CHOKING, For Unconscious Infant Under 1 Year.

DON'TS

- Don't give chest compressions if there is a heartbeat; doing so may cause the heart to stop beating.

- If you suspect a spinal injury, don't move your infant's head or neck to check for breathing.

WHEN TO GET PROFESSIONAL HELP

- If you are not alone, have one person call your local emergency number immediately while another person begins CPR.

- If you are alone, shout for help! If you are trained in CPR, administer CPR for about 1 minute, then call your local emergency number.

- If you are alone and not trained in CPR, call your local emergency number immediately—emergency personnel will tell you what to do.

1. Rub your infant's back or tap her shoulder to determine whether she is conscious.

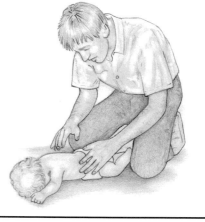

2. If she doesn't respond, turn her on her back as a unit onto a hard surface, keeping her back in a straight line, firmly supporting her head and neck. Expose her chest.

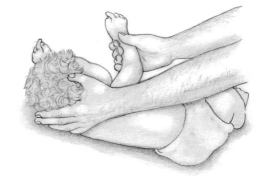

CONTINUED ON NEXT PAGE |||▶

3. Lift your infant's chin while tilting her head back to move her tongue away from her windpipe.

If you suspect a spinal injury, pull her jaw forward without moving her head or neck. Don't let her mouth close.

4. Place your ear close to your infant's mouth and watch for chest movement. For 5 seconds, look, listen, and feel for breathing.

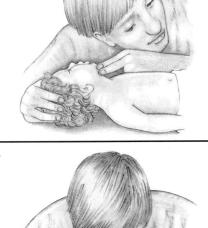

5. If she is not breathing, begin rescue breathing, as follows:

Maintain her head position and cover her mouth and nose tightly with your mouth. Give 2 slow, gentle breaths, each lasting 1 second with a pause in between.

6. If you don't see her chest rise, reposition her head and give 2 more breaths.

If her chest still doesn't rise, her airway is obstructed. Turn to page 30—CHOKING, For Unconscious Infant Under 1 Year.

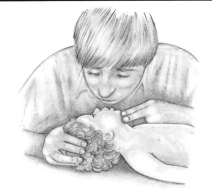

CONTINUED ON NEXT PAGE

7. If you do see your infant's chest rise, place 2 fingers on the inside of her upper arm, just above the elbow. Squeeze gently to feel her pulse for 5 to 10 seconds.

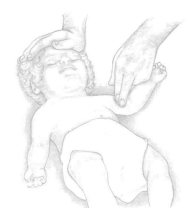

8. If she has a pulse, give 1 breath every 3 seconds. Check her pulse after every 20 breaths.

After 1 minute, call your local emergency number. Resume giving breaths and checking the pulse.

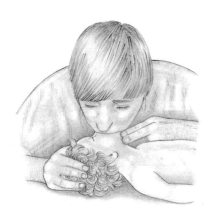

9. If your infant has no pulse, begin chest compressions, as follows:

Maintain her head position and place 2 fingers on the middle of her breastbone, just below her nipples. Within 3 seconds, quickly press your fingers ½ to 1 inch (1¼ to 2½ cm) into her chest 5 times. Give the compressions in a smooth, rhythmic manner, keeping your fingers on her chest.

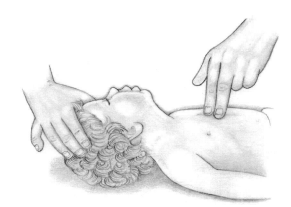

CONTINUED ON NEXT PAGE |||⟩

10. Give your infant 1 breath, followed by 5 chest compressions. Repeat this sequence 10 times.

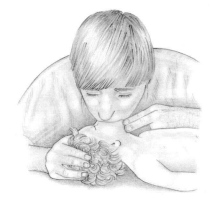

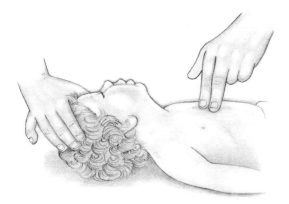

11. Recheck her pulse for 5 to 10 seconds.

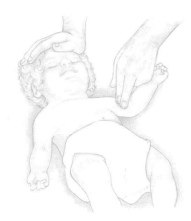

12. Repeat Steps 10 and 11 until your infant's pulse resumes or help arrives. If her pulse resumes, go to Step 8.

16 Breathing/Cardiac Emergency **For Child Age 1–8 Years**

WHAT YOU NEED TO KNOW

- The procedures for CPR (cardiopulmonary resuscitation) described below are not a substitute for CPR training; they are performed most effectively and safely by those trained in CPR.

- If choking is the cause of breathing difficulty, follow the procedures on page 36—CHOKING, For Unconscious Child Over 1 Year.

DON'TS

- Don't give chest compressions if there is a heartbeat; doing so may cause the heart to stop beating.

- If you suspect a spinal injury, don't move your child's head or neck to check for breathing.

WHEN TO GET PROFESSIONAL HELP

- If you are not alone, have one person call your local emergency number immediately while another person begins CPR.

- If you are alone, shout for help! If you are trained in CPR, administer CPR for about 1 minute, then call your local emergency number.

- If you are alone and not trained in CPR, call your local emergency number immediately—emergency personnel will tell you what to do.

---

1. Tap or shake your child gently and call his name to determine consciousness.

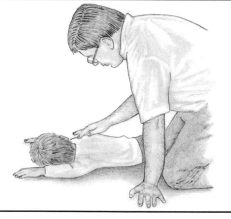

---

2. If he doesn't respond, turn him on his back as a unit onto a hard surface, keeping his back in a straight line, firmly supporting his head and neck. Expose his chest.

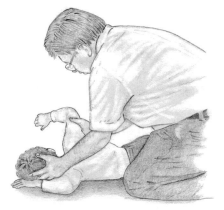

CONTINUED ON NEXT PAGE ||||➡

3. **Lift your child's chin while tilting his head back to move his tongue away from his windpipe.**

If you suspect a spinal injury, pull his jaw forward without moving his head or neck. Don't let his mouth close.

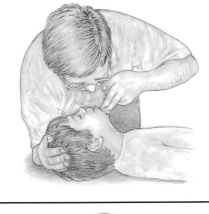

4. **Place your ear close to your child's mouth and watch for chest movement. For 5 seconds, look, listen, and feel for breathing.**

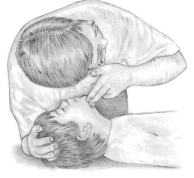

5. **If he is not breathing, begin rescue breathing, as follows:**

Maintain his head position, close his nostrils by pinching them with your thumb and index finger, and cover his mouth tightly with your mouth. Give 2 slow, full breaths, with a pause in between.

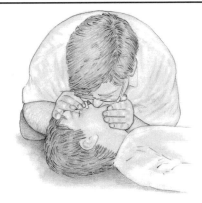

6. **If you don't see his chest rise, reposition his head and give 2 more breaths.**

If his chest still doesn't rise, his airway is obstructed. Turn to page 36—CHOKING, For Unconscious Child Over 1 Year.

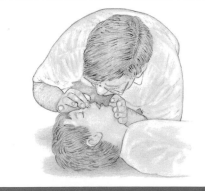

CONTINUED ON NEXT PAGE |||||➤

7. **If you do see your child's chest rise, place 2 fingers on his Adam's apple. Slide your fingers into the groove between the Adam's apple and the muscle on the side of his neck to feel his pulse for 5 to 10 seconds.**

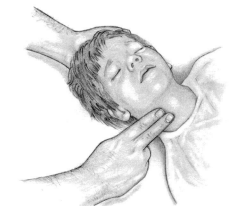

8. **If he has a pulse, give 1 breath every 4 seconds. Check his pulse after every 15 breaths.**

After 1 minute, call your local emergency number. Resume giving breaths and checking the pulse.

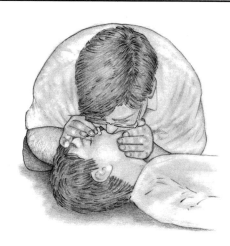

9. **If your child has no pulse, begin chest compressions, as follows:**

Maintain his head position and place the heel of your hand 2 finger-widths above the lowest notch of his breastbone. Lean your shoulders over your hand, and within 4 seconds quickly press down 1 to 1½ inches (2½ to 4 cm) into his chest 5 times. Give the compressions in a smooth, rhythmic manner, keeping your hand on his chest.

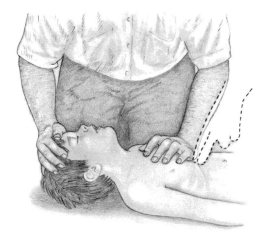

CONTINUED ON NEXT PAGE ⟫➡

10. Give your child 1 breath, followed by 5 chest compressions. Repeat this sequence 10 times.

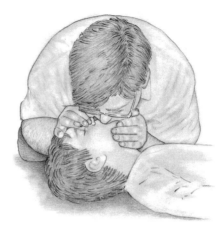

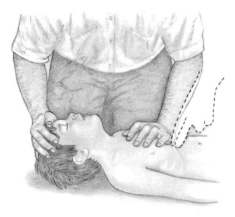

11. Recheck his pulse for 5 to 10 seconds.

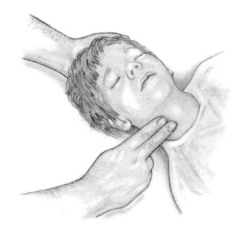

12. Repeat Steps 10 and 11 until your child's pulse resumes or help arrives. If his pulse resumes, go to Step 8.

WHAT YOU NEED TO KNOW

- The procedures for CPR (cardiopulmonary resuscitation) described below are not a substitute for CPR training; they are performed most effectively and safely by those trained in CPR.

- If choking is the cause of breathing difficulty, follow the procedures on page 36—CHOKING, For Unconscious Child Over 1 Year.

DON'TS

- Don't give chest compressions if there is a heartbeat; doing so may cause the heart to stop beating.

- If you suspect a spinal injury, don't move your child's head or neck to check for breathing.

WHEN TO GET PROFESSIONAL HELP

- If you are not alone, have one person call your local emergency number immediately while another person begins CPR.

- If you are alone, shout for help! If you are trained in CPR, administer CPR for about 1 minute, then call your local emergency number.

- If you are alone and not trained in CPR, call your local emergency number immediately—emergency personnel will tell you what to do.

---

1. Tap or shake your child gently and call her name to determine consciousness.

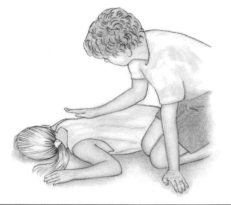

---

2. If she doesn't respond, turn her on her back as a unit onto a hard surface, keeping her back in a straight line, firmly supporting her head and neck. Expose her chest.

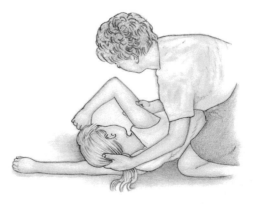

CONTINUED ON NEXT PAGE ⫸

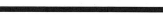

3. Lift your child's chin while tilting her head back to move her tongue away from her windpipe.

If you suspect a spinal injury, pull her jaw forward without moving her head and neck. Don't let her mouth close.

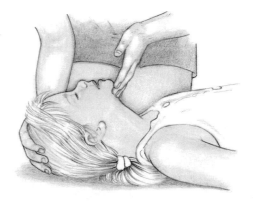

4. Place your ear close to your child's mouth and watch for chest movement. For 5 seconds, look, listen, and feel for breathing.

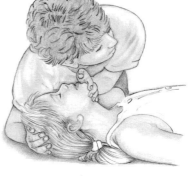

5. If she is not breathing, begin rescue breathing, as follows:

Maintain her head position, close her nostrils by pinching them with your thumb and index finger, and cover her mouth tightly with your mouth. Give 2 slow, full breaths, with a pause in between.

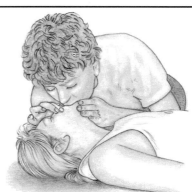

6. If you don't see her chest rise, reposition her head and give 2 more breaths.

If her chest still doesn't rise, her airway is obstructed. Turn to page 36—CHOKING, For Unconscious Child Over 1 Year.

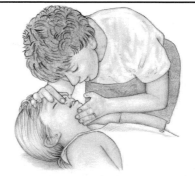

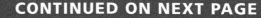
CONTINUED ON NEXT PAGE

7. If you do see your child's chest rise, place 2 fingers on her Adam's apple. Slide your fingers into the groove between the Adam's apple and the muscle on the side of her neck to feel her pulse for 5 to 10 seconds.

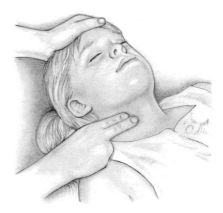

8. If she has a pulse, give 1 breath every 5 seconds. Check her pulse after every 12 breaths.

After 1 minute, call your local emergency number. Resume giving breaths and checking the pulse.

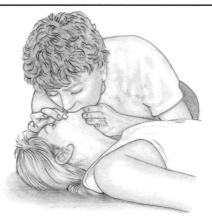

9. If your child has no pulse, begin chest compressions, as follows:

Maintain her head position and place the heel of your hand 2 finger-widths above the lowest notch of her breastbone. Place the heel of your other hand directly over the heel of the first hand. Interlock your fingers; don't let them touch your child's chest. Lean your shoulders over your hands, and within 10 seconds quickly press down 1½ to 2 inches (4 to 5 cm) into her chest 15 times. Give the compressions in a smooth, rhythmic manner, keeping your hands on her chest.

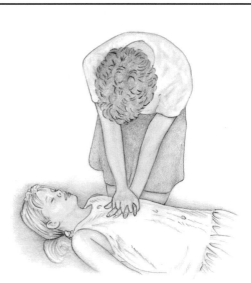

CONTINUED ON NEXT PAGE ||||➡

10. Give your child 2 breaths, followed by 15 chest compressions. Repeat this sequence 4 times.

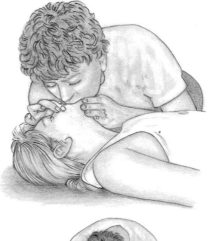

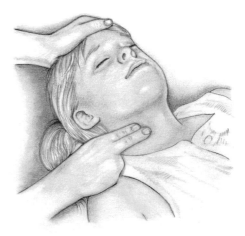

11. Recheck her pulse for 5 to 10 seconds.

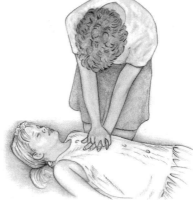

12. Repeat Steps 10 and 11 until your child's pulse resumes or help arrives. If her pulse resumes, go to Step 8.

24 Burns

SIGNS & SYMPTOMS

- *First-degree* burns affect the outer layer of the skin, causing pain, redness, and swelling.
- *Second-degree* burns affect both the outer and underlying layer of the skin, causing pain, redness, swelling, and blistering.
- *Third-degree* burns extend into deeper tissues, causing brown or blackened skin that may be numb.

WHAT TO CHECK

- If the burn is extensive, observe your child for shock. If the child becomes dizzy or faint and/or develops pale, cool, clammy skin; rapid, shallow breathing; and a weak, rapid pulse, turn to page 80—SHOCK.

WHEN TO GET PROFESSIONAL HELP

- If the burn is extensive, call your local emergency number.
- For any chemical or electrical burn, or if you are uncertain about the burn's severity, call your doctor.

DON'TS

- Don't remove dead skin or break blisters.
- Don't apply ice, butter, ointments, medications, fluffy cotton dressings, or adhesive bandages to a burn.

1. **If your child has a *chemical burn*, immediately remove all burned clothing and immerse the burned area in cool water under a tap or hose—or, if burns are extensive, place your child in a shower or bathtub—for 10 minutes.**

Pat dry. Go to Step 4.

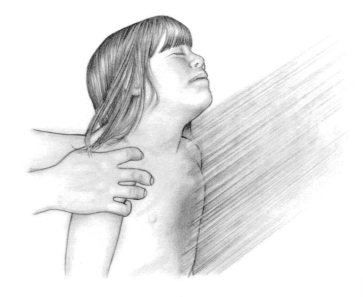

CONTINUED ON NEXT PAGE ⫸

2. **If your child is *on fire*, either (a) douse her with water if it is available; (b) wrap her in thick, nonsynthetic material such as a wool or cotton coat, rug, or blanket to smother the flames; or (c) lay her flat and roll her on the ground.**

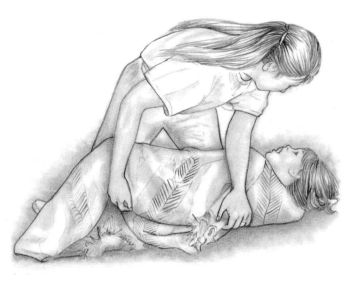

If your clothes catch fire, STOP, DROP, AND ROLL. When the fire is out, go to Step 3.

3. **If your child has a *heat, fire, or electrical burn,* remove any clothing that comes off easily and rinse the burned area in cool water under a shower, tap, or hose, depending on the extent of the burn, until the pain subsides.**

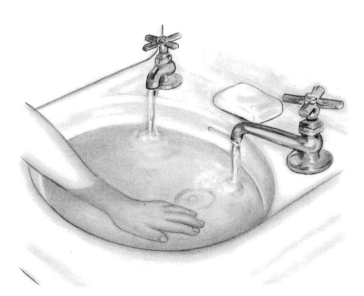

Cover burned areas that cannot be immersed, such as the face, with wet cloths. Pat dry.

CONTINUED ON NEXT PAGE ⫸

4. Cover the burned area with a clean, dry, nonfluffy dressing.

If the burn is on your child's hands or feet, keep her fingers or toes apart by placing cloth or gauze between them; then loosely wrap the hand or foot in a clean dressing.

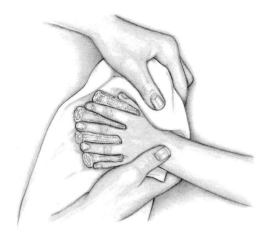

5. If the burn is minor, over the next 24 to 48 hours observe the wound for signs of infection (increasing redness, swelling, and pain).

If the burn becomes infected, call your doctor or take your child to an emergency facility.

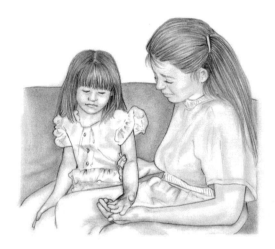

6. If the burn is extensive and your child is not vomiting, give her liquids to help replace lost fluids.

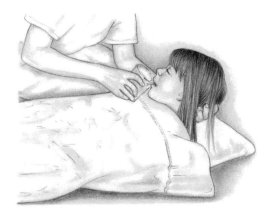

SIGNS & SYMPTOMS

- Inability to breathe or cry; high-pitched noises; ineffective coughs; face begins to turn blue.

WHEN TO GET PROFESSIONAL HELP

- If you are not alone, have one person call your local emergency number while another person follows the first aid steps below.

- If you are alone and can do so quickly, call your local emergency number. Then follow the first aid steps below.

- Even if you successfully dislodge the obstruction and your infant seems fine, call your doctor for further instructions.

DON'TS

- Don't interfere with your infant if he can still cough, breathe, or cry.

- Don't try to grasp the object lodged in your infant's throat; you may push it farther down.

- If breathing has stopped, don't begin CPR until the airway is cleared.

- Don't initiate the first aid steps below until you are certain your infant is actually choking. If he can't cough or cry, or his coughing and crying is very weak, then follow the first aid steps below.

1. Lay your infant face down along your forearm with his chest in your hand and his jaw between your thumb and index finger. Use your thigh or lap for support. Keep his head lower than his body.

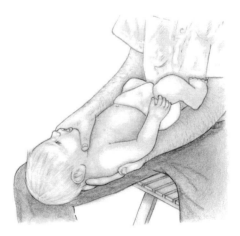

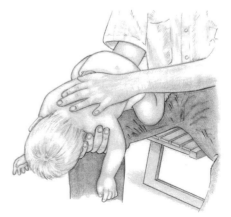

CONTINUED ON NEXT PAGE ⫘➡

2. **Within 5 seconds, give 4 quick, forceful blows between his shoulder blades with the heel of your other hand.**

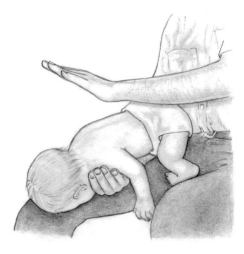

3. **Turn your infant over so he is face up on your other arm. Use your thigh or lap for support. Keep his head lower than his body.**

4. **Place 2 fingers on the middle of his breastbone just below his nipples.**

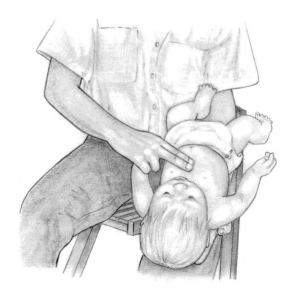

CONTINUED ON NEXT PAGE ||||⇒

5. Within 1 second, quickly thrust your fingers ½ to 1 inch (1¼ to 2½ cm) into his chest 4 times.

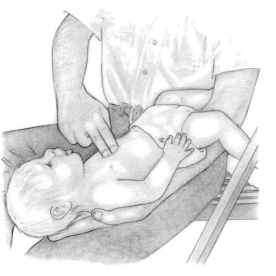

6. Turn your infant over so he is face down on your other arm and give another 4 back blows. Continue alternating 4 back blows with 4 chest thrusts until the object is dislodged, help arrives, or your infant loses consciousness.

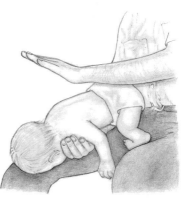

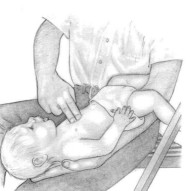

If your infant loses consciousness, turn to the next page—CHOKING, For Unconscious Infant Under 1 Year.

WHAT TO CHECK

- Rub your infant's back or tap his shoulder to determine whether he is conscious. If he doesn't respond, then follow the first aid steps below.

DON'TS

- Don't try to grasp the object lodged in your infant's throat; you may push it farther down.

- If breathing has stopped, don't begin CPR until the airway is cleared.

WHEN TO GET PROFESSIONAL HELP

- If you are not alone, have one person call your local emergency number while another person follows the first aid steps below.

- If you are alone, shout for help! If you can do so quickly, call your local emergency number. Then follow the first aid steps below.

- Even if you successfully dislodge the obstruction and your infant seems fine, call your doctor for further instructions.

---

1. Firmly supporting your infant's head and neck, place him on his back as a unit onto a hard surface, keeping his back in a straight line. Expose his chest.

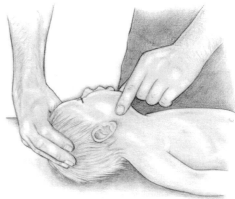

---

2. Open your infant's mouth with your thumb and index finger, placing your thumb over his tongue. *If the object is visible and loose, remove it.*

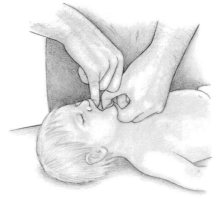

CONTINUED ON NEXT PAGE

3. Look, listen, and feel for breathing.

Lift your infant's chin while tilting his head back to move his tongue away from his windpipe. Don't let his mouth close. Place your ear close to his mouth and watch for chest movement. For 5 seconds, look, listen, and feel for breathing.

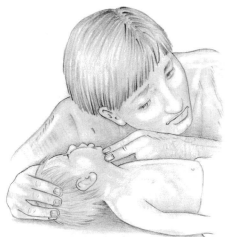

4. If your infant is not breathing, begin rescue breathing, as follows:

Maintain his head position and cover his mouth and nose tightly with your mouth. Give 2 slow, gentle breaths, each lasting 1 second with a pause in between.

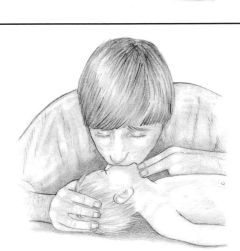

5. If you don't see his chest rise, reposition his head and give 2 more breaths.

CONTINUED ON NEXT PAGE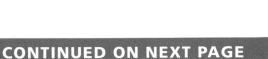

6. If your infant's chest still doesn't rise, begin back blows.

Lay him face down along your forearm with his chest in your hand and his jaw between your thumb and index finger. Use your thigh or lap for support. Keep his head lower than his body.

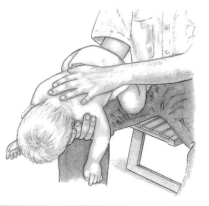

7. Within 5 seconds, give 4 quick, forceful blows between his shoulder blades with the heel of your other hand.

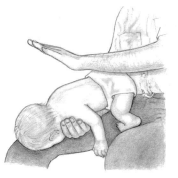

8. Turn your infant over so he is face up on your other arm. Use your thigh or lap for support. Keep his head lower than his body.

9. Place 2 fingers on the middle of his breastbone just below his nipples.

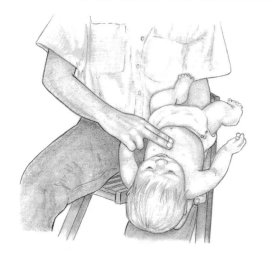

CONTINUED ON NEXT PAGE ||||⇒

10. Within 1 second, quickly thrust your fingers ½ to 1 inch (1¼ to 2½ cm) into his chest 4 times.

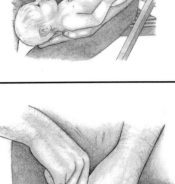

11. Open your infant's mouth with your thumb and index finger, placing your thumb over his tongue. *If the object is visible and loose,* remove it. Observe his breathing.

If your infant stops breathing, begin CPR (see page 12—BREATHING/ CARDIAC EMERGENCY, For Infant Under 1 Year).

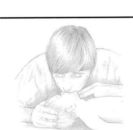

12. If the object is not dislodged, give 2 breaths, 4 back blows, 4 chest thrusts, and then check for the object. Repeat this sequence until the object is dislodged or help arrives.

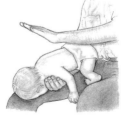

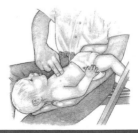

SIGNS & SYMPTOMS

- Inability to breathe, talk, or cry; high-pitched noises; ineffective coughs; face begins to turn blue.

WHEN TO GET PROFESSIONAL HELP

- If you are not alone, have one person call your local emergency number while another person follows the first aid steps below.

- If you are alone and can do so quickly, call your local emergency number. Then follow the first aid steps below.

- Even if you successfully dislodge the obstruction and your child seems fine, call your doctor for further instructions.

DON'TS

- Don't interfere with your child if she can still cough, breathe, talk, or cry.

- Don't try to grasp the object lodged in your child's throat; you may push it farther down.

- If breathing has stopped, don't begin CPR until the airway is cleared.

- Don't initiate the first aid steps below until you are certain your child is actually choking. Encourage coughing to clear the airway. If she can't cough or her cough is very weak, then follow the first aid steps below.

1. **Stand behind your child and wrap your arms around her waist.**

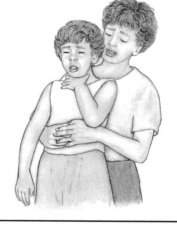

2. **Make a fist with your hand. Grasp the fist with your other hand. Place the thumb-side of your fist in the middle of your child's abdomen, just above the navel and well below the tip of her breastbone.**

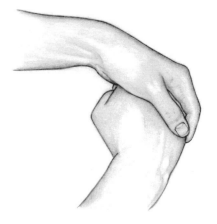

CONTINUED ON NEXT PAGE

3. Keep your elbows out and press your fist into your child's abdomen inward and upward with quick, distinct thrusts.

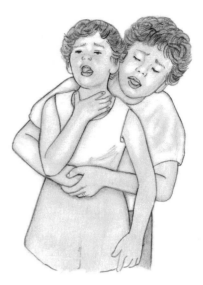

4. Continue these abdominal thrusts until the object is dislodged, help arrives, or your child loses consciousness.

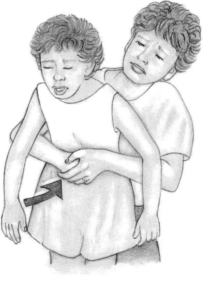

If your child loses consciousness, turn to the next page—CHOKING, For Unconscious Child Over 1 Year.

WHAT TO CHECK

- Tap or shake your child gently and call her name to determine whether she is conscious. If she doesn't respond, then follow the first aid steps below.

DON'TS

- Don't try to grasp the object lodged in your child's throat; you may push it farther down.

- If breathing has stopped, don't begin CPR until the airway is cleared.

WHEN TO GET PROFESSIONAL HELP

- If you are not alone, have one person call your local emergency number while another person follows the first aid steps below.

- If you are alone, shout for help! If you can do so quickly, call your local emergency number. Then follow the first aid steps below.

- Even if you successfully dislodge the obstruction and your child seems fine, call your doctor for further instructions.

1. Firmly supporting your infant's head and neck, place her on her back as a unit onto a hard surface, keeping her back in a straight line. Expose her chest.

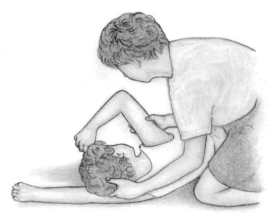

2. Open your child's mouth with your thumb and index finger, placing your thumb over her tongue. *If the object is visible and loose, remove it.*

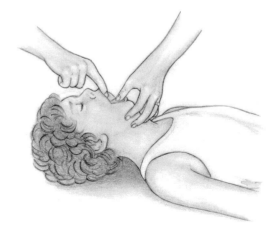

CONTINUED ON NEXT PAGE ⁞⁞⁞➡

3. Look, listen, and feel for breathing.

Lift your child's chin while tilting her head back to move her tongue away from her windpipe. Don't let her mouth close. Place your ear close to her mouth and watch for chest movement. For 5 seconds, look, listen, and feel for breathing.

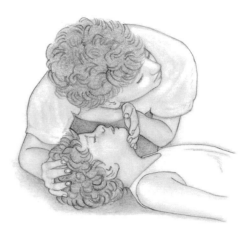

4. If your child is not breathing, begin rescue breathing, as follows:

Maintain her head position, close her nostrils by pinching them with your thumb and index finger, and cover her mouth tightly with your mouth. Give 2 slow, full breaths, with a pause in between.

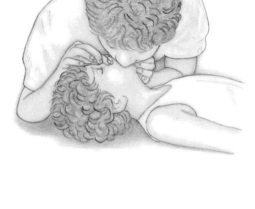

5. If you don't see her chest rise, reposition her head and give 2 more breaths.

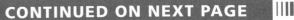

CONTINUED ON NEXT PAGE ⫸

6. If your child's chest still doesn't rise, begin abdominal thrusts, as follows:

Kneel at her feet or astride her thighs. Place the heel of your hand in the middle of her abdomen just above her navel, well below the tip of her breastbone. Place your other hand on top of the first hand.

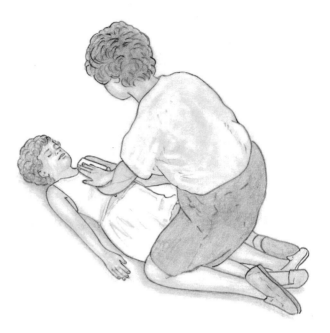

7. Press into your child's abdomen with 6 to 10 quick, continuous upward thrusts.

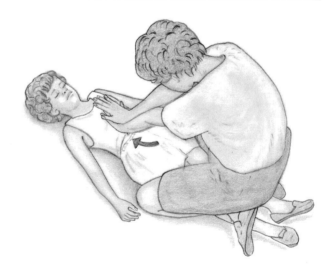

CONTINUED ON NEXT PAGE ⫸

8. **Open your child's mouth with your thumb and index finger. *If the object is visible and loose, remove it. Observe her breathing.***

If your child stops breathing, begin CPR:

If your child is 1 to 8 years old, see page 16—BREATHING/CARDIAC EMERGENCY, For Child Age 1–8 Years.

If your child is over 8 years old, see page 20—BREATHING/CARDIAC EMERGENCY, For Child Over 8 Years.

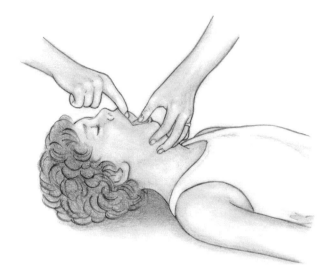

9. **If the object is not dislodged, give 2 breaths, 6 to 10 abdominal thrusts, and then check for the object. Repeat this sequence until the object is dislodged or help arrives.**

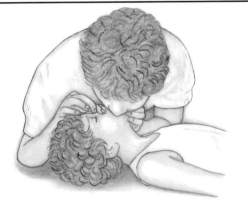

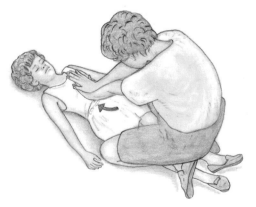

SIGNS & SYMPTOMS

- Numbness, pain and burning, hard skin, yellowish white or bluish white skin, blisters.

WHAT YOU NEED TO KNOW

- Frostbite most frequently affects exposed areas, such as the fingers, toes, ears, nose, and cheeks.

WHAT TO CHECK

- Your child may also have hypothermia. If the child is shivering uncontrollably, turn immediately to page 42—COLD EMERGENCIES, Hypothermia.

WHEN TO GET PROFESSIONAL HELP

- If you think that the cold exposure was prolonged, call your doctor or take your child to an emergency facility.

DON'TS

- Don't treat affected parts with hot water or a dry heat source such as a hair dryer or space heater.

- Don't rub or massage affected parts or break blisters.

- Don't thaw affected parts if you are outdoors and refreezing could occur.

1. **Take your child indoors as soon as possible, remove wet clothing from the affected area, and remove any rings from frostbitten hands.**

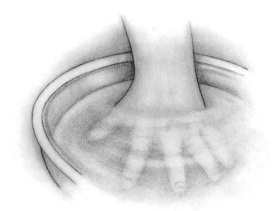

2. **Immerse affected areas in warm (not hot) water—or apply warm cloths to affected ears, nose, or cheeks—for 20 to 30 minutes.**

Add water as needed to maintain water temperature. Your child will probably complain of intense pain as thawing progresses. After thawing, pat affected parts dry.

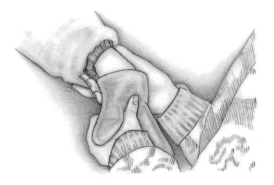

CONTINUED ON NEXT PAGE ⫸

- **If feeling and color return, no further treatment is needed.**

- **If feeling and color do not return, call your doctor and continue with Steps 3 through 5.**

3. Wrap affected hands or feet loosely in a clean dressing.

Keep fingers or toes apart by placing cloth or gauze between them before wrapping the hand or foot. Be careful not to break blisters by rubbing.

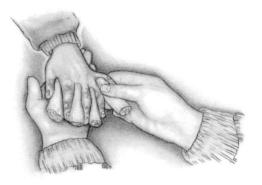

4. Elevate affected hands or feet.

Have your child try to move the affected parts to increase circulation. Don't let him walk if his feet are affected.

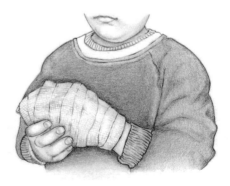

5. If the frostbite is extensive, give your child warm liquids to replace lost fluids.

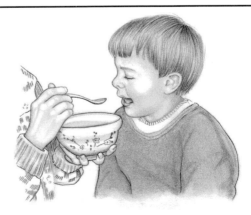

SIGNS & SYMPTOMS

- Uncontrollable shivering, weakness, drowsiness, confusion, slowing of breathing, or shock.

- Very low body temperature—less than 95°F (35°C).

WHAT YOU NEED TO KNOW

- Bodies lose heat much faster in cold water or through wet clothing than when dry.

WHAT TO CHECK

- Observe your child for shock. If the child becomes dizzy or faint and/or develops pale, cool, clammy skin; rapid, shallow breathing; and a weak, rapid pulse, turn to page 80—SHOCK.

WHEN TO GET PROFESSIONAL HELP

- If you observe the signs and symptoms listed above, if your child's temperature is less than 95°F (35°C), or if you think that cold exposure was prolonged, call your local emergency number.

1. Bring your child into a warm room (if in the woods, start a fire and create shelter from the wind), remove any wet clothing, and keep her awake.

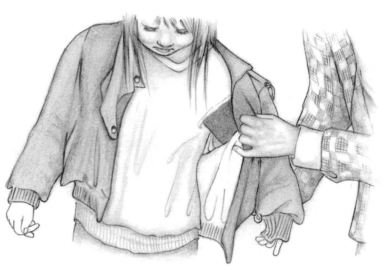

CONTINUED ON NEXT PAGE |||⟩

2. Wrap your child in warm blankets or clothing and cover her head; then apply heat to her torso with hot-water bottles or heating pads, and/or warm her with body-to-body contact.

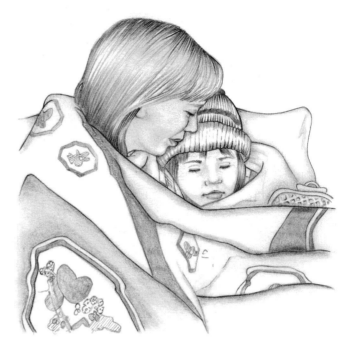

3. If your child is conscious, give her warm liquids.

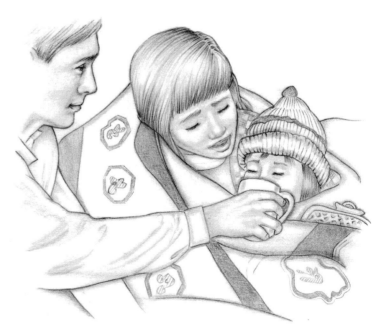

44 Convulsion/Seizure

- Uncontrollable body movements, eyes rolling back, foaming at the mouth, loss of bowel and bladder control, loss of consciousness.

WHAT YOU NEED TO KNOW

- Remain calm; most convulsions stop within 5 to 10 minutes.

- Many childhood convulsions are caused by fever (especially if there is a rapid increase in temperature) and are not serious. Seizures that are not prolonged (over 30 to 45 minutes) do not cause brain damage.

WHEN TO GET PROFESSIONAL HELP

- If the convulsion lasts more than 10 minutes, call your local emergency number.

- If the convulsion is your child's first, or if your child has more than one convulsion, call your doctor.

DON'TS

- Don't restrain your child, try to force his mouth open, and/or try to grasp his tongue.

---

1. If necessary, move your child to a safe place where he cannot be injured.

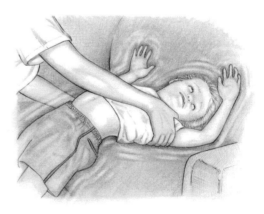

---

2. Stay with your child unless you need to obtain medical help.

Loosen his clothing at the neck and the waist.

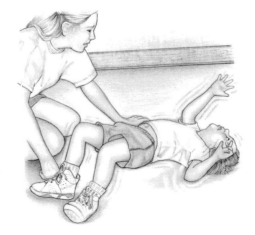

CONTINUED ON NEXT PAGE

3. Place your child on his side to prevent him from choking if he vomits.

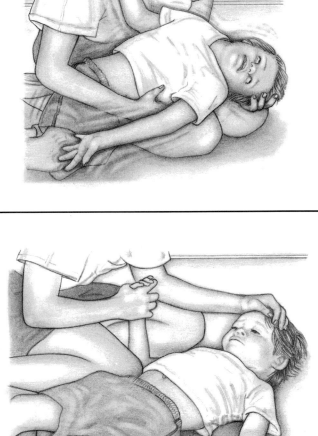

4. If the convulsion has stopped and your child feels feverish, turn to page 63—FEVER.

WHEN TO GET PROFESSIONAL HELP

- If possible, call your local emergency number immediately.

- After an ice rescue, if your child is unconscious, if he has been submerged for any period of time, if he is hypothermic (see page 42—COLD EMERGENCIES, Hypothermia), or if you have any concerns, call your local emergency number; otherwise call your doctor.

DON'TS

- Don't go out on the ice to rescue a child you can reach with your arm or an extended object.

- Don't let a drowning child grab you; he might pull you under.

WHAT YOU NEED TO KNOW

- With ice rescue, time is of the essence. Submersion in ice water can rapidly cause hypothermia.

- Give CPR if needed, even to a child who has been submerged for an extended period. Continue CPR until help arrives or your child begins to breathe on his own.

  If your child is under 1 year old, see page 12—BREATHING/CARDIAC EMERGENCY, For Infant Under 1 Year.

  If your child is 1 to 8 years old, see page 16—BREATHING/CARDIAC EMERGENCY, For Child Age 1–8 Years.

  If your child is over 8 years old, see page 20—BREATHING/CARDIAC EMERGENCY, For Child Over 8 Years.

1. Have your child extend his arms flat on the ice and kick to keep afloat.

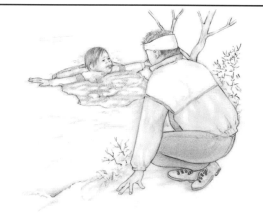

2. Kneel or lie down near the edge of the ice, brace yourself firmly, and reach for your child with your arm or an extended object such as a stick, a rope, or clothing.

If you must move onto the ice, lie flat and edge out slowly until the extended object is within the child's reach.

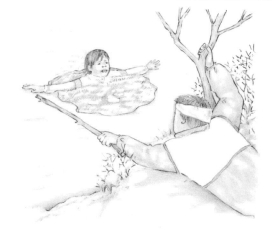

CONTINUED ON NEXT PAGE ‖‖➡

3. **Have your child lie flat while you pull him to safety; don't let him get up and walk off the ice.**

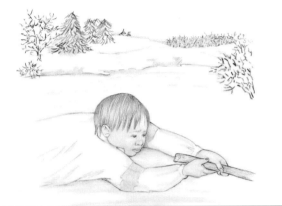

4. **If you can't pull your child out with an extended object and other people are available, form a human chain to pull him out.**

Have everyone slide out on the ice lying flat and spread-eagled, grasping the ankles of the person in front.

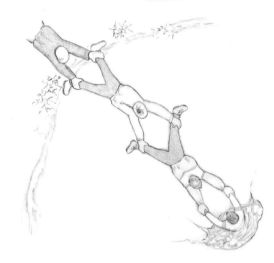

5. **Observe your child's breathing, check the pulse, and give CPR if needed.**

If your child is under 1 year old, see page 12— BREATHING/CARDIAC EMERGENCY, For Infant Under 1 Year.

If your child is 1 to 8 years old, see page 16— BREATHING/CARDIAC EMERGENCY, For Child Age 1–8 Years.

If your child is over 8 years old, see page 20— BREATHING/CARDIAC EMERGENCY, For Child Over 8 Years.

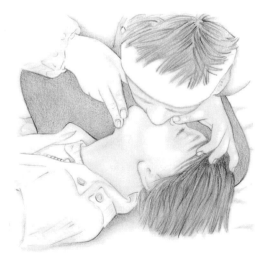

CONTINUED ON NEXT PAGE ||||➡

6. **If your child vomits, turn his head to the side and remove the vomitus from his mouth.**

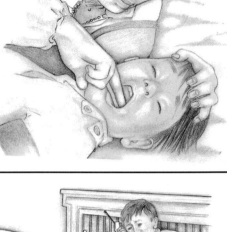

7. **If your child is breathing, take him to a warm place, remove any wet clothing, wrap him in blankets, and call for professional help.**

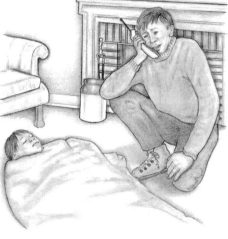

8. **If your child is shivering uncontrollably, call your local emergency number and treat him for possible hypothermia.**

Turn to page 42—COLD EMERGENCIES, Hypothermia.

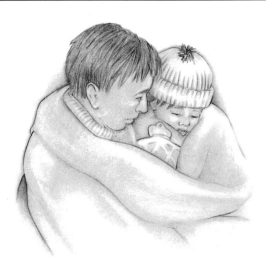

WHEN TO GET PROFESSIONAL HELP

- If possible, call your local emergency number immediately.

- After a water rescue, if your child is unconscious, if she has been submerged for any period of time, or if you have any concerns, call your local emergency number; otherwise call your doctor.

DON'TS

- Don't enter the water to rescue a child who can be reached with your arm, a boat, an extended object, or a throwable object.

- Don't let a drowning child grab you; she might pull you under.

WHAT YOU NEED TO KNOW

- A child who is drowning often cannot call out for help.

- Give CPR if needed, even to a child who has been submerged for an extended period, especially in cold water. Continue CPR until help arrives or your child begins to breathe on her own.

  If your child is under 1 year old, see page 12—BREATHING/CARDIAC EMERGENCY, For Infant Under 1 Year.

  If your child is 1 to 8 years old, see page 16—BREATHING/CARDIAC EMERGENCY, For Child Age 1–8 Years.

  If your child is over 8 years old, see page 20—BREATHING/CARDIAC EMERGENCY, For Child Over 8 Years.

1. If your child is within reach, kneel or lie down near the edge of the water, brace yourself firmly, and reach for her with your arm or an extended object such as a pole, oar, or towel.

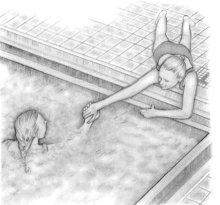

2. If your child is beyond reach, throw a buoyant object such as a board or a life ring to her.

If possible, throw an object with a line attached so you can pull her in; try to throw the object past her and then pull it within her reach. If the object has no line, tell her to grab the object and kick to safety.

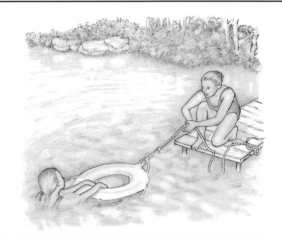

CONTINUED ON NEXT PAGE ⫸

3. If your child is beyond reach, wade into the water if it is safe to do so, and extend an object to her.

Either pull her to safety or, if the object is buoyant, let go of it and tell her to kick to safety. Be sure to keep the object between you and the child—don't let her grab you.

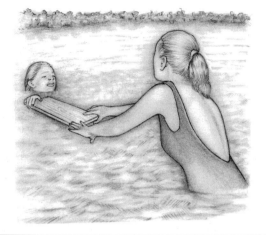

4. If you must swim to your child, keep your eye on the spot where you last saw her and bring an object for her to hold on to—don't let her grab you.

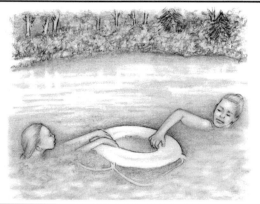

5. If your child is not breathing, begin mouth-to-mouth resuscitation—while still in the water if possible. Once on land, check the pulse and give CPR if needed.

If your child is under 1 year old, see page 12— BREATHING/CARDIAC EMERGENCY, For Infant Under 1 Year.

If your child is 1 to 8 years old, see page 16— BREATHING/CARDIAC EMERGENCY, For Child Age 1–8 Years.

If your child is over 8 years old, see page 20— BREATHING/CARDIAC EMERGENCY, For Child Over 8 Years.

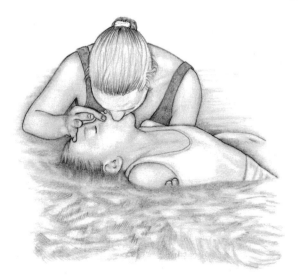

CONTINUED ON NEXT PAGE ‖‖‖⇒

6. **If your child vomits, turn her head to the side and remove the vomitus from her mouth.**

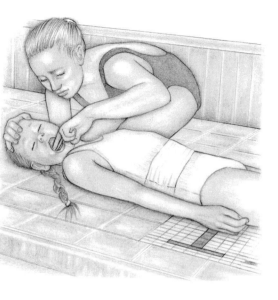

7. **If your child is breathing, remove any wet clothing, wrap her in blankets, and call for professional help.**

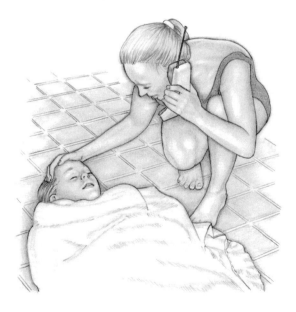

52 Earache

- Pain, irritability, prolonged or excessive crying, dizziness, ringing in ear, discharge, hearing loss.

WHAT YOU NEED TO KNOW

- Ear infections are very common in infancy and childhood and are often associated with colds.

WHEN TO GET PROFESSIONAL HELP

- If your child has an earache, call your doctor. All ear infections, even mild ones, require treatment.

1. Give your child pain-relieving tablets or liquid (acetaminophen or paracetamol).

Follow the dosage recommended on the package label.

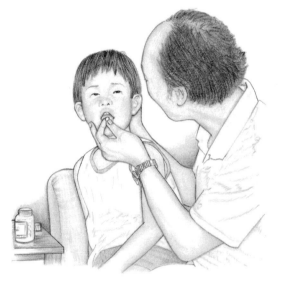

2. If previously prescribed, give your child eardrops for pain.

Warm the bottle in your hand and lay the child on his back with his head turned to the side. Pull his ear up and out, and insert 3 or 4 drops in the ear canal. Place a small piece of cotton in his ear if tolerated. Keep him lying down with his head turned to the side for a few minutes to allow drops to come in contact with the eardrum.

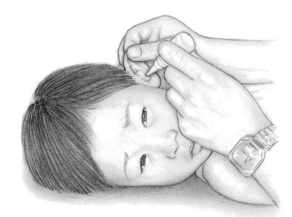

CONTINUED ON NEXT PAGE

3. **Apply a heating pad or hot-water bottle to the ear to reduce discomfort.**

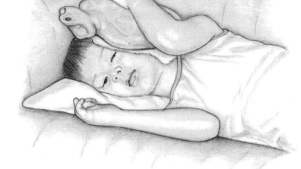

4. **If your child is uncomfortable lying down, let him rest in an upright position to reduce pressure in the middle ear.**

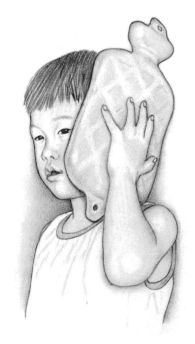

WHAT YOU NEED TO KNOW

- An electrical shock may be brief and harmless, or it may be life threatening.

WHEN TO GET PROFESSIONAL HELP

- If your child is unconscious, has difficulty breathing, or has extensive electrical burns, call your local emergency number.
- If your child has electrical burns, which are often more severe than they seem, call your doctor.

DON'TS

- Don't touch your child with your bare hands while she is still in contact with the source of electricity.
- If burns are present, don't remove dead skin or break blisters.
- Don't apply ice, butter, ointments, medications, fluffy cotton dressings, or adhesive bandages to a burn.

WHAT TO CHECK

- Observe your child for signs of shock. If the child becomes dizzy or faint and/or develops pale, cool, clammy skin; rapid, shallow breathing; and a weak, rapid pulse, turn to page 80—SHOCK.
- Observe your child's breathing and check the pulse. If needed, begin CPR:

   If your child is under 1 year old, see page 12—BREATHING/CARDIAC EMERGENCY, For Infant Under 1 Year.

   If your child is 1 to 8 years old, see page 16—BREATHING/CARDIAC EMERGENCY, For Child Age 1–8 Years.

   If your child is over 8 years old, see page 20—BREATHING/CARDIAC EMERGENCY, For Child Over 8 Years.

1. Unplug the cord or remove the fuse from the fuse box to turn off the electric current.

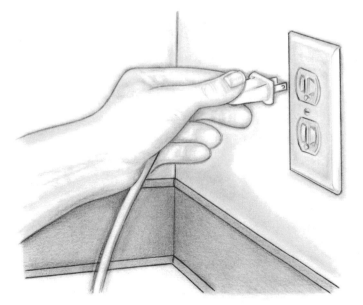

CONTINUED ON NEXT PAGE ⅢⅢ➡

2. **If the current can't be turned off, use a nonconducting object such as a broom, chair, rug, or rubber doormat to push your child away from the source of the current.**

Don't use a wet or metal object. If possible, stand on something dry and nonconducting, such as a mat or folded newspapers.

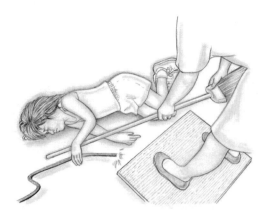

3. **If your child has an electrical burn, remove any clothing that comes off easily and rinse the burned area in cool running water until the pain subsides.**

Cover burned areas that cannot be immersed, such as the face, with wet cloths. Pat dry.

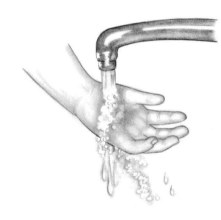

4. **If the burn is still painful, cover the burned area with a clean, dry, nonfluffy dressing.**

If the burn is on your child's hands or feet, keep her fingers or toes apart by placing cloth or gauze between them; then loosely wrap the hand or foot in a clean dressing.

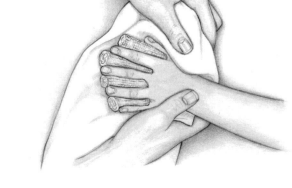

- Prompt flushing of the eye is important.

- If any chemicals get in your child's eye, call your doctor or take your child to an emergency facility.

1. Turn your child's head so the injured eye is down and to the side. Holding the eyelid open, use a cup or a shower-head to pour water in the eye for 15 minutes (or use sterile eye wash).

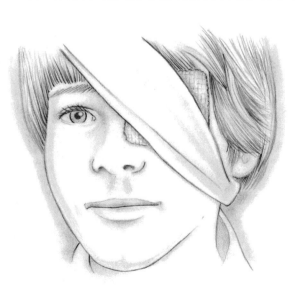

2. Cover the injured eye with a clean dressing, and don't let your child rub his eye.

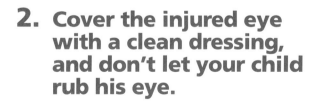

SIGNS & SYMPTOMS

- **Constant blinking of the eyes, light sensitivity, pain.**

DON'TS

- **Don't apply pressure to the cornea (the outer covering of the eyeball).**

- **Don't let your child touch her eye.**

WHEN TO GET PROFESSIONAL HELP

- **If your child's cornea is scratched, call your doctor or take your child to an emergency facility for a definitive diagnosis and medication, if needed.**

1. **Cover both eyes with a clean dressing for 24 to 48 hours.**

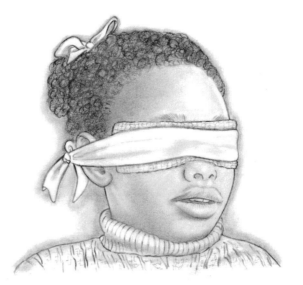

- If the cut is large or turns black and blue, call your doctor or take your child to an emergency facility; a tear duct or nerve may be injured, which requires professional treatment.

1. If the cut is bleeding, apply direct pressure with a clean, dry cloth until the bleeding subsides.

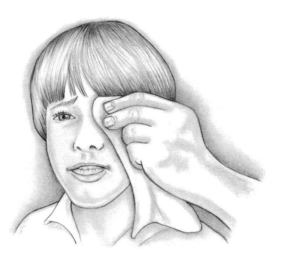

2. Clean the cut with water, cover with a clean dressing, and place a cold compress on the dressing to reduce pain and swelling.

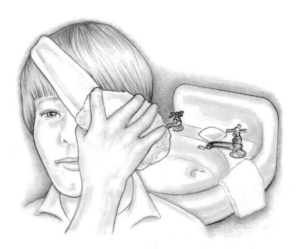

WHEN TO GET PROFESSIONAL HELP

- If you cannot remove the foreign object (dirt, sand, etc.), call your doctor or take your child to an emergency facility.

DON'TS

- Don't try to remove a foreign object that seems to be embedded in the eye.
- Don't use sharp objects such as tweezers to remove the object.

1. Grasp the top eyelid and pull it out and down over the eye.

The object may wash out with tears.

2. Gently depress the lower eyelid and look for the object.

If you see the object, carefully lift it off with a clean cloth or, if your child is cooperative, a cotton swab.

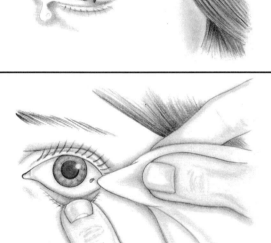

3. Have your child blink, which may force the object out.

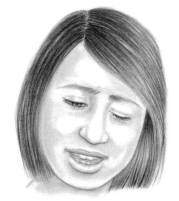

CONTINUED ON NEXT PAGE

4. **Grasp the top eyelid and turn it back over a cotton swab.**

Have your child look down. Remove the object with a clean cloth or by flushing the eye with water or sterile eye wash.

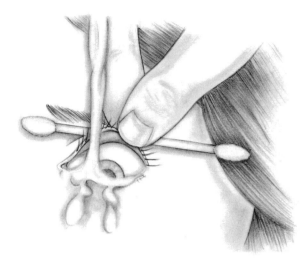

5. **If the object cannot be removed, cover the eye with a clean dressing and call your doctor or take your child to an emergency facility.**

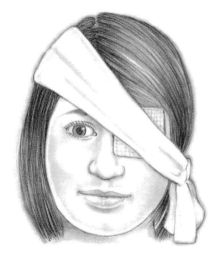

SIGNS & SYMPTOMS

- Pallor, dizziness, sweating, passing out.

WHAT TO CHECK

- If your child remains unconscious, observe breathing and check the pulse. If needed, begin CPR:

  If your child is under 1 year old, see page 12—BREATHING/CARDIAC EMERGENCY, For Infant Under 1 Year.

  If your child is 1 to 8 years old, see page 16—BREATHING/CARDIAC EMERGENCY, For Child Age 1–8 Years.

  If your child is over 8 years old, see page 20—BREATHING/CARDIAC EMERGENCY, For Child Over 8 Years.

WHEN TO GET PROFESSIONAL HELP

- If your child does not regain consciousness after 5 minutes, call your local emergency number.

DON'TS

- Don't splash water on your child's face, shake him, or use smelling salts.

---

1. If your child becomes light-headed, place his head between his knees.

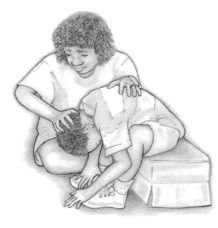

---

2. Loosen your child's clothing and make sure he has sufficient air.

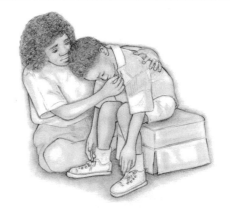

CONTINUED ON NEXT PAGE |||||➡

3. **If your child loses consciousness, place him on his back and elevate his feet 8 to 12 inches (20 to 30 cm).**

Don't place a pillow under your child's head.

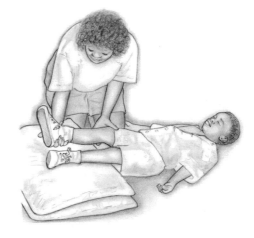

4. **Turn your child's head to the side to prevent him from choking if he vomits.**

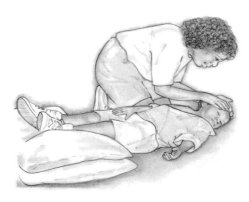

5. **Wait 5 to 10 minutes after your child regains consciousness before allowing him to stand or walk.**

If he fell, check for any injuries. If you suspect significant injuries, especially to the head, call your doctor immediately.

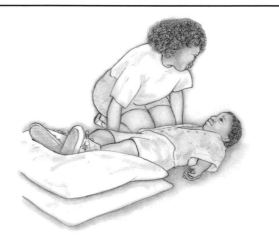

WHAT YOU NEED TO KNOW

- Many infants and children develop high fevers, even with minor viral illnesses.

- Fevers below 106°F (41°C) do not cause brain damage.

WHEN TO GET PROFESSIONAL HELP

- If an infant under 3 or 4 months has a temperature above 101°F (38.5°C), or if a child of any age has a fever above 103°F (39.5°C) for more than 24 hours that is not associated with other symptoms, call your doctor.

DON'TS

- Don't use ice water or rubbing alcohol to reduce your child's temperature.

- Don't bundle a feverish child in blankets.

- Don't wake a sleeping child to give her medication or take her temperature; sleep is more important.

1. **If your child's temperature is over 102°F (39°C), or if she is uncomfortable, give her pain-relieving tablets or liquid (acetaminophen or paracetamol).**

Follow the dosage recommended on the package label.

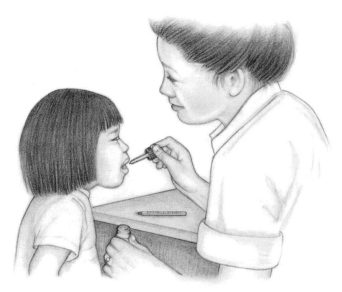

CONTINUED ON NEXT PAGE

2. If your child's temperature is over 103.5°F (40°C) 1 to 2 hours after giving her medication for fever, place her in a tub of lukewarm water up to her navel.

Rub a wet washcloth or towel over your child's body for 20 minutes or for as long as she will tolerate it. Add warm water as needed to maintain the water temperature and keep her from shivering. Pat (don't rub) her dry.

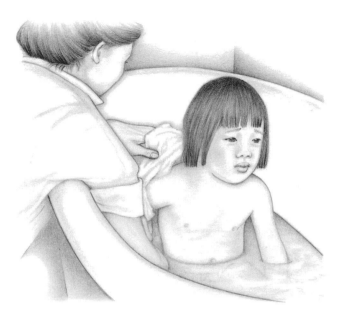

3. Dress your child in light clothing, give her liquids, and keep the room comfortably cool.

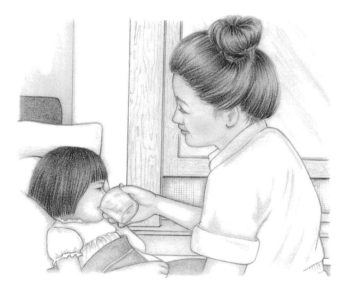

SIGNS & SYMPTOMS

- Pain, swelling, bruising, deformity, limitation of movement, pain on weight bearing.

WHAT YOU NEED TO KNOW

- A fracture is the cracking, breaking, or buckling of bones; a dislocation is the displacement or slippage of bones from joints.

- Always immobilize a fractured or dislocated part in the position in which it was found.

WHAT TO CHECK

- If there is bleeding, observe your child for signs of shock. If he becomes dizzy or faint and/or develops pale, cool, clammy skin; rapid, shallow breathing; and a weak, rapid pulse, continue to treat the bleeding and turn to page 80—SHOCK.

WHEN TO GET PROFESSIONAL HELP

- If you suspect an injury to the spine, a severe head injury, or multiple fractures, or if a chest injury is associated with difficulty breathing, call your local emergency number.

- If your child has a fracture or dislocation, call your doctor or take the child to an emergency facility.

DON'TS

- If you suspect a spinal injury or a broken hip, pelvis, or thigh, don't move your child unless absolutely necessary. If you must move him, see Step 6 below.

- Don't try to move or reposition a fractured or dislocated part.

1. Treat any bleeding with direct pressure.

Turn to page 10—BLEEDING. Cover the wound with a clean dressing.

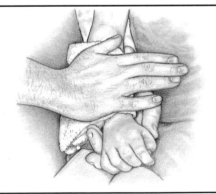

2. If the injury is to the shoulder or upper arm, immobilize the arm with a triangular cloth sling and tie the sling to the body.

Turn to page viii—HOW TO MAKE A SLING.

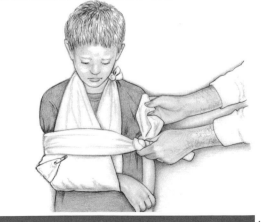

CONTINUED ON NEXT PAGE |||||▶

3. **If the injury is to a limb or finger, immobilize the injured part—in the position in which it was found—with a padded splint.**

Turn to page vii—HOW TO MAKE A SPLINT.

If the injury is to a forearm, after splinting it, place the arm in a triangular cloth sling and tie the sling to the body. Turn to page viii—HOW TO MAKE A SLING.

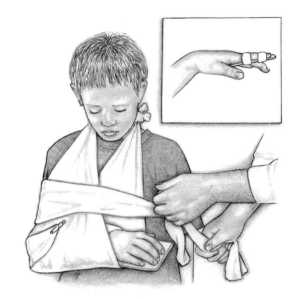

4. **If the injury is to the hip, pelvis, or thigh, and you are waiting for an ambulance, immobilize the injured area by placing rolled-up towels, blankets, or clothing between your child's legs.**

Don't let your child move his legs.

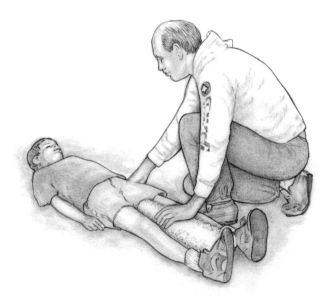

CONTINUED ON NEXT PAGE IIII➡

5. **If the injury is to the hip, pelvis, or thigh, and you must move your child yourself, immobilize the injured part on a stretcher.**

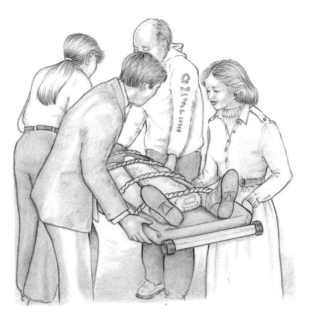

If possible, get several people to help. Use a sturdy board such as an ironing board or another long, flat object that extends from the child's head to his heels. Together, roll his entire body as a unit—keeping the head, neck, and back in a straight line—toward you. Slide the board alongside him. Roll him onto the board, again keeping the head and torso stable. Place rolled-up towels, blankets, or clothing between his legs. Use ropes, belts, tape, or strips of cloth to help hold him in place on the stretcher. Keep him as horizontal as possible when transporting him.

6. **If your child is uncomfortable, apply a cold compress to the injury to reduce pain and swelling.**

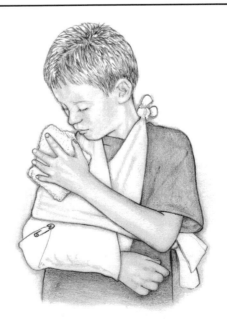

SIGNS & SYMPTOMS

- *Minor head injury:* lump or cut on the head, brief period of vomiting, brief loss of consciousness and confusion or double vision, occasionally 1 to 2 hours of drowsiness.

- *Serious head injury:* lump or cut on the head, persistent vomiting, extended period of unconsciousness, amnesia, confusion or double vision, drowsiness, convulsions, clear or bloody nasal discharge, inability to respond to simple questions or commands or to move uninjured body parts, initial improvement followed by worsening symptoms.

WHAT YOU NEED TO KNOW

- The signs and symptoms of a head injury may occur immediately or develop slowly over several hours.

WHEN TO GET PROFESSIONAL HELP

- If your child shows any of the signs and symptoms of a *serious* head injury, call your local emergency number.

- If your child shows any of the signs or symptoms of a *minor* head injury, call your doctor.

DON'TS

- Don't move your child if you suspect a serious head injury or a spinal injury (see page 81—SPINAL INJURY).

- If your child is wearing a helmet and you suspect a serious head injury, don't remove the helmet.

- Don't wash a head wound that is deep or bleeding profusely.

1. Attempt to stop any bleeding by firmly pressing a clean cloth on the wound.

If the injury is serious, be careful not to move your child's head. If blood soaks through the cloth, don't remove it; you may loosen the clot. Place another cloth over the first one.

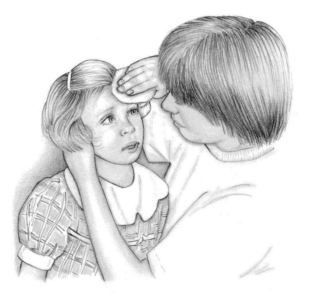

CONTINUED ON NEXT PAGE |||⏢➡

2. **If the head wound is superficial, wash it with soap and warm water and pat dry.**

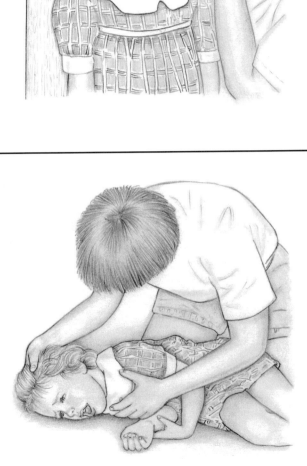

3. **If your child is vomiting and you don't suspect a spinal injury, turn her head to the side to prevent her from choking.**

If you suspect a spinal injury, get several people to help, if possible, and together try to roll your child's entire body as a unit—keeping head, neck, and back in a straight line—toward you onto her side.

CONTINUED ON NEXT PAGE |||||➡

4. If there is swelling and pain, apply a cold compress to the injury and give your child pain-relieving tablets or liquid (acetaminophen or paracetamol).

Follow the dosage recommended on the package label.

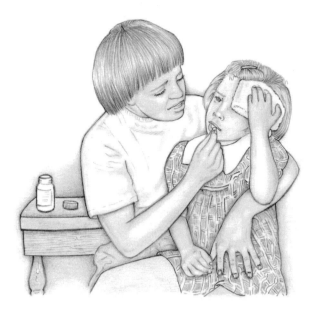

5. Over the next 12 to 24 hours, observe your child for any signs and symptoms of a serious head injury.

During the night, wake your child every 1 to 2 hours. If she cannot respond to simple questions or commands, or if vomiting persists, call your doctor or take the child to an emergency facility.

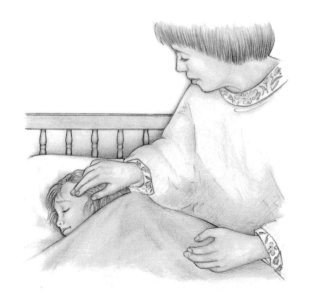

SIGNS & SYMPTOMS

- Fatigue, nausea, dizziness, profuse sweating, thirst (temperature remains normal or slightly elevated).

WHAT TO CHECK

- Take your child's temperature. If your child has a high temperature—102 to 106°F (39 to 41°C)—and is not sweating, he may have heat stroke, which can be very serious. Turn immediately to page 72—HEAT EMERGENCIES, Heat Stroke. If his temperature is normal or slightly elevated, follow the first aid steps below.

WHEN TO GET PROFESSIONAL HELP

- If your child's temperature is high—102 to 106°F (39 to 41°C)—call your local emergency number.

- If your child's temperature is above 101°F (38.5°C), or if signs and symptoms last longer than 1 to 2 hours or worsen, call your doctor.

1. **Remove your child from sunlight and have him lie down in a cool place.**

Loosen his clothing.

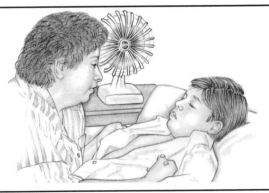

2. **Unless your child is vomiting, have him sip water or juices every 10 to 15 minutes.**

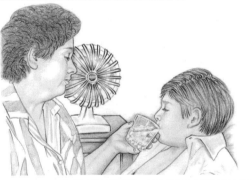

3. **Apply cool, wet cloths to your child's skin and fan him.**

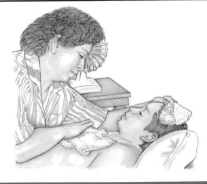

SIGNS & SYMPTOMS

- Absence of sweating; hot, flushed skin; headache; dizziness; confusion; nausea/vomiting; muscle cramps; bounding or weak and rapid pulse; loss of consciousness; high temperature—102 to 106°F (39 to 41°C).

WHAT TO CHECK

- Observe your child for signs of shock. If she becomes dizzy or faint and/or develops pale, cool, clammy skin; rapid, shallow breathing; and a weak, rapid pulse, turn to page 80—SHOCK.

WHEN TO GET PROFESSIONAL HELP

- If you suspect heat stroke, call your local emergency number and immediately try to lower your child's body temperature; heat stroke can be very serious.

DON'TS

- Don't give your child medications or stimulants such as caffeinated soft drinks.

1. Remove your child from direct sunlight, and begin a cool-down procedure.

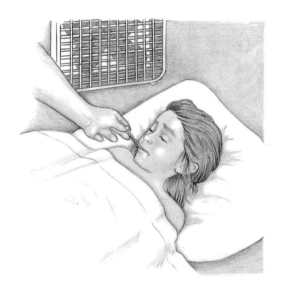

Do one of the following:
- (a) place her in a tub of cool (not cold) water up to her navel and rub a wet washcloth or towel over her body,
- (b) put her in a cool shower or under a garden hose, or
- (c) lay her down in a cool room in front of a fan or air conditioner and wrap her in wet sheets or towels.

Continue cooling her until her temperature drops to 102°F (39°C) or lower.

2. When your child's temperature has dropped to 102°F (39°C), pat her dry, lay her down, and cover her with a dry sheet.

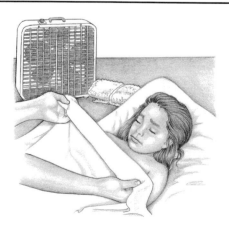

Fan her or put her in front of a fan or air conditioner. If her temperature begins to rise, repeat Step 1.

- Dry air, blowing or picking the nose frequently, and blows to the nose cause most nosebleeds.

- If bleeding persists after 15 to 20 minutes of treatment, nosebleeds recur, or blood persistently drains down your child's throat, call your doctor.

1. Calm and reassure your child.

Bleeding will be less severe if she relaxes.

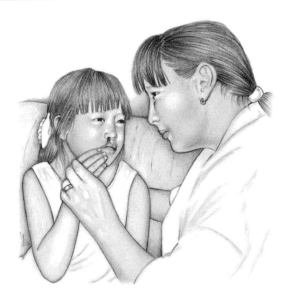

2. Have your child lean forward and pinch her nose shut for at least 10 minutes to allow a blood clot to form.

Don't let her sniff or blow her nose for several hours. If the bleeding persists or recurs, repeat Step 2.

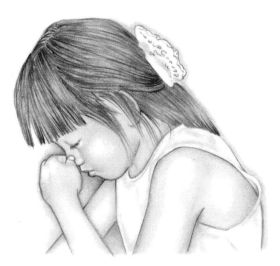

CONTINUED ON NEXT PAGE ⫼⮕

3. After bleeding stops, gently apply petroleum jelly to the inside of the nostrils with a cotton swab to prevent drying.

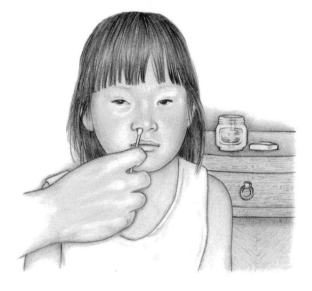

4. If the air in your child's bedroom is dry, using a cool-mist vaporizer may help prevent nosebleeds from recurring.

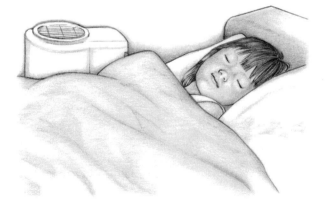

SIGNS & SYMPTOMS

- Bleeding, difficulty breathing, a visible foreign object in the nose, foul-smelling discharge from the nostrils (especially from one nostril).

WHAT YOU NEED TO KNOW

- Small children often put foreign objects in their nose.

WHEN TO GET PROFESSIONAL HELP

- If you can't easily remove the object, call your doctor or take your child to an emergency facility.

DON'TS

- Don't try to remove an object that is not visible and easy to grasp; doing so may push the object farther in and/or damage tissue.

1. If the object is visible and easy to grasp, try to remove it with your fingers or round-ended tweezers.

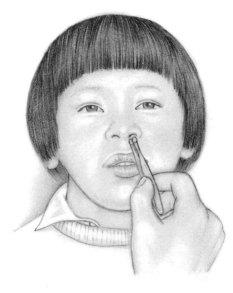

2. If the object can't be removed, have your child blow his nose if he is able to do so.

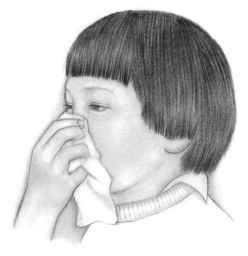

SIGNS & SYMPTOMS

- Swelling, redness, pain, bleeding.

WHAT YOU NEED TO KNOW

- Bruising under the eyes may occur after a day or two.

WHEN TO GET PROFESSIONAL HELP

- If (a) the pain is severe or persists after treatment, (b) the bleeding cannot be controlled or recurs, (c) the nose seems misshapen, or (d) breathing through each nostril separately is difficult, call your doctor.

- Very few nose injuries cause problems requiring immediate professional attention. The doctor may prefer to see your child after the swelling subsides.

1. Calm and reassure your child.

Bleeding and swelling will be less severe if she relaxes.

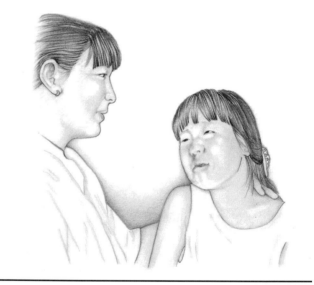

2. Stop bleeding as you would for a nosebleed.

Turn to page 73—NOSE EMERGENCIES, Bleeding.

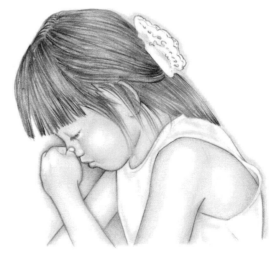

CONTINUED ON NEXT PAGE |||||➡

3. Apply cold compresses to the nose to reduce swelling.

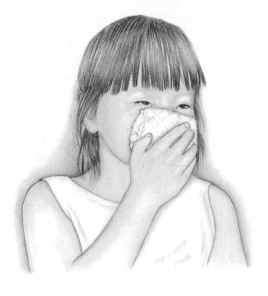

4. Give your child pain-relieving tablets or liquid (acetaminophen or paracetamol), if needed.

Follow the dosage recommended on the package label.

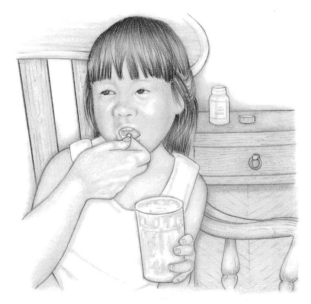

SIGNS & SYMPTOMS

- Sudden onset of illness or change in behavior, which may take many forms depending on the substance ingested.

WHAT YOU NEED TO KNOW

- Poisoning can be serious, but frequently can be managed at home. Prompt determination of the substance ingested and immediate treatment are essential.

- Medicines, cleaning fluids, and houseplants are the most common causes of poisoning.

- If possible, bring samples of the ingested substance and/or the vomitus with you to the hospital for analysis.

WHAT TO CHECK

- Observe your child's breathing and check the pulse. If needed, begin CPR:

  If your child is under 1 year old, see page 12—BREATHING/CARDIAC EMERGENCY, For Infant Under 1 Year.

  If your child is 1 to 8 years old, see page 16—BREATHING/CARDIAC EMERGENCY, For Child Age 1–8 Years.

  If your child is over 8 years old, see page 20—BREATHING/CARDIAC EMERGENCY, For Child Over 8 Years.

WHEN TO GET PROFESSIONAL HELP

- If your child is unconscious and/or has difficulty breathing, call your local emergency number.

- Otherwise call your local or regional Poison Control Center, doctor, or hospital immediately for instructions.

- Don't induce vomiting if your child has swallowed a caustic substance such as drain cleaner or disinfectant, or a petroleum product such as gasoline or lighter fluid.

1. If your child is conscious, try to determine what he swallowed.

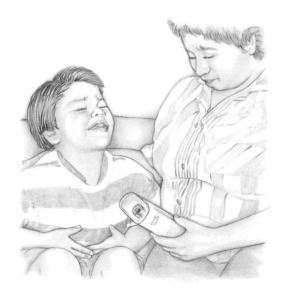

CONTINUED ON NEXT PAGE

2. If instructions from the Poison Control Center, doctor, or hospital aren't available and your child has not swallowed a caustic substance or a petroleum product, give him 1 tablespoon (15 ml) of syrup of ipecac followed by 2 glasses of water to induce vomiting.

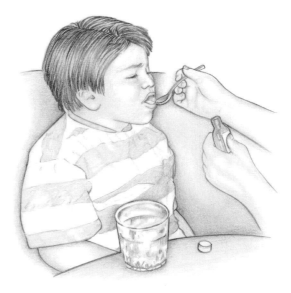

3. For any swallowed liquid (not pills), give your child 2 to 3 glasses of water to dilute the liquid.

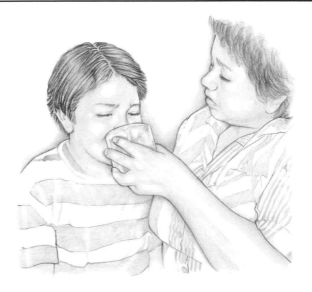

80 Shock

- Pale, cool, clammy skin; dizziness/faintness; thirst; nausea/vomiting; rapid, shallow breathing; weak, rapid pulse.

WHAT YOU NEED TO KNOW

- Shock may result from injuries with extensive blood loss, a severe allergic reaction, a serious infection, or heart disease.

- If shock results from blood loss, stop the bleeding before treating the shock.

DON'TS

- If you suspect spinal injury, don't move your child.

- If your child vomits, don't give her anything to eat or drink.

WHAT TO CHECK

- Observe your child's breathing and check the pulse. If needed, begin CPR:

  If your child is under 1 year old, see page 12—BREATHING/CARDIAC EMERGENCY, For Infant Under 1 Year.

  If your child is 1 to 8 years old, see page 16—BREATHING/CARDIAC EMERGENCY, For Child Age 1–8 Years.

  If your child is over 8 years old, see page 20—BREATHING/CARDIAC EMERGENCY, For Child Over 8 Years.

WHEN TO GET PROFESSIONAL HELP

- If you suspect shock, call your local emergency number. Shock requires immediate treatment to prevent damage to vital organs and tissues.

1. If your child is conscious and doesn't have a head or chest injury with difficulty breathing, place her on her back and elevate her feet 8 to 12 inches (20 to 30 cm).

If your child is conscious and has a head or chest injury or difficulty breathing, elevate her head but *not* her feet.

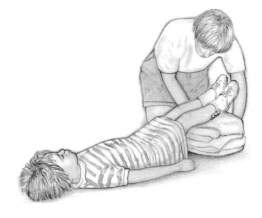

2. Cover your child with a blanket or jacket to keep her warm.

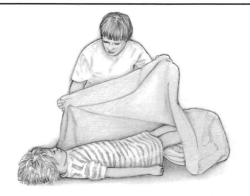

SIGNS & SYMPTOMS

- Stiff neck, head held in unusual position, weakness, paralysis of extremities, difficulty walking, shock, and the signs associated with a serious head injury (turn to page 68—HEAD INJURIES).

WHEN TO GET PROFESSIONAL HELP

- If the injury is to the back or neck, call your local emergency number immediately.

DON'TS

- Don't bend, twist, or lift your child's head or body.
- Don't attempt to move your child before medical help arrives. If he must be moved, see Step 5 below.
- If your child is wearing a helmet, don't remove it.

1. If your child is unconscious, check for breathing.

Without moving or lifting your child's neck or head, pull the jaw forward to open the airway. Make sure the tongue is not obstructing the airway. Look, listen, and feel for breathing.

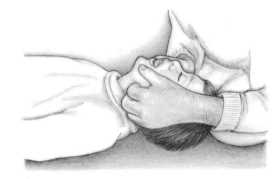

If he is breathing, go to Step 3.

2. If your child isn't breathing, begin CPR.

Follow the CPR directions:

If your child is under 1 year old, see page 12—BREATHING/CARDIAC EMERGENCY, For Infant Under 1 Year.

If your child is 1 to 8 years old, see page 16—BREATHING/CARDIAC EMERGENCY, For Child Age 1–8 Years.

If your child is over 8 years old, see page 20—BREATHING/CARDIAC EMERGENCY, For Child Over 8 Years.

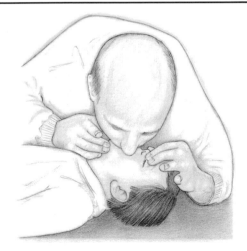

When he resumes regular breathing, go to Step 3. Continue to observe breathing and check the pulse.

CONTINUED ON NEXT PAGE ||||➡

3. Immobilize your child's head and torso in the position found.

Place rolled-up towels, clothing, or blankets around his head and torso. If your child is on his back, slide a pad or small towel under his neck without moving his head. Make sure his collar is loose. Keep supports in place with heavy objects such as books or stones. If possible, tape his forehead as shown.

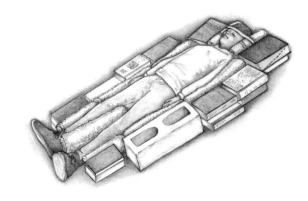

If emergency personnel are on the way, no further treatment is needed.

4. If you must move your child, get several people to help.

Use a sturdy support, such as an ironing board or a plank, as a stretcher. Together, roll your child's entire body as a unit— keeping head, neck, and back in a straight line—toward you. Slide the board alongside the child. Roll him onto the board, keeping the head and torso stable.

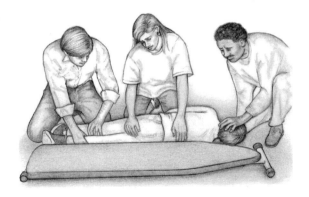

5. Immobilize your child's head and torso in the position found.

Place rolled-up towels, clothing, or blankets around his head and torso. Use ropes, belts, tape, or strips of cloth to hold him in place on the stretcher. Carry the stretcher as horizontally as possible.

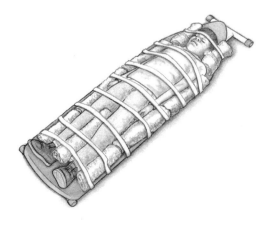

SIGNS & SYMPTOMS

- Pain, swelling, cramping or stiffness, limitation of joint mobility, bruising.

WHAT YOU NEED TO KNOW

- A *sprain* is the tearing and/or stretching of a ligament; a *strain* is the tearing and/or stretching of a muscle or tendon.

- If you suspect a fracture, turn to page 65—FRACTURES & DISLOCATIONS.

WHEN TO GET PROFESSIONAL HELP

- If (a) the pain or swelling is severe, (b) your child's ability to move the affected area is limited, (c) a bone is deformed and possibly broken, (d) the injured area remains painful after 48 hours, or (e) your child is unable to apply pressure to the injured area after 48 hours, call your doctor.

1. **Have your child rest in a comfortable position.**

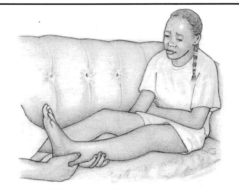

2. **If possible, elevate the injured area above heart level to slow blood flow and reduce swelling.**

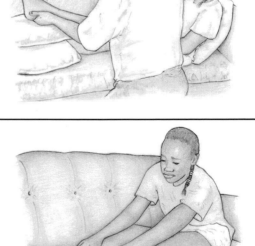

3. **Apply a cold compress to the injured area for 10 to 15 minutes to reduce swelling and pain.**

If swelling persists, reapply the cold compress every 20 to 30 minutes until the swelling decreases.

CONTINUED ON NEXT PAGE |||▶

4. Give your child pain-relieving tablets or liquid (acetaminophen or paracetamol), if needed.

Follow the dosage recommended on the package label.

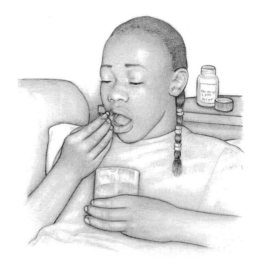

5. If your child has an injury to the leg, ankle, or knee, bandage the affected area firmly but not tightly.

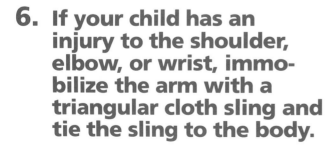

6. If your child has an injury to the shoulder, elbow, or wrist, immobilize the arm with a triangular cloth sling and tie the sling to the body.

Turn to page viii—HOW TO MAKE A SLING.

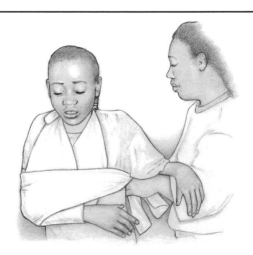

CONTINUED ON NEXT PAGE |||||➡

7. After 48 hours, if pain and swelling have decreased, have your child try to move the affected joint in all directions.

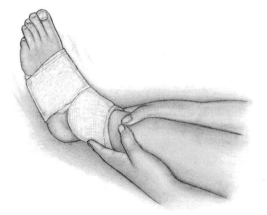

8. Keep pressure off the injured area until the pain subsides, usually 7 to 10 days for mild sprains and strains and 4 to 6 weeks for severe sprains and strains.

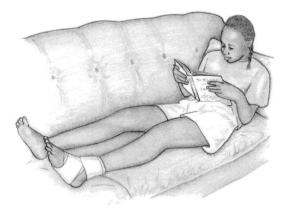

Parents' Emergency Information Page

LOCAL EMERGENCY PHONE: _____

DOCTOR OR CLINIC:

Name _____

Phone _____

Address _____

HOSPITAL:

Name _____

Phone _____

Address _____

Directions to Hospital _____

_____

_____

_____

POISON CONTROL CENTER: _____

FIRE: _____

POLICE: _____

ANIMAL CONTROL OR VETERINARIAN: _____

NEIGHBOR OR RELATIVE:

Name _____

Phone _____

MOTHER'S PHONE AT WORK: _____

FATHER'S PHONE AT WORK: _____